MEDITERRANEAN DIET FOR BEGINNERS

Complete beginners guide for easy mediterranean home recipes

TABLE OF CONTENTS

INTRODUCTION

Did you know that there is a lifestyle and way of eating that can actually make you look and feel younger as well as help you reduce your risk of chronic diseases and maintain healthy body weight? It's living the Mediterranean way—eating a diet rich in foods like fish, whole grains, fresh fruits and vegetables and heart-healthy fats like olive oil. Research on the benefits of the Mediterranean diet has caused experts to shine a light on the healthy, and proven, lifestyle practices of this region. "The more closely you adhere to the Mediterranean diet, the lower your chance of having disease or disability, the lower your chance of having a health event like a heart attack, and the younger your Real Age. So while you're enjoying delicious foods such as grilled fish or a tomato and cucumber salad, you'll know that you're making yourself younger." Luckily, you don't have to relocate or even visit the Mediterranean region to realize healthful results. All you have to do is introduce a few simple habits into your own life. Cook and eat fresh, whole foods, slow down to enjoy the flavors and stay active.

There exist an overwhelming number of diets that have been introduced to the world to date. Every diet promises results only minutely dissimilar from the next, and it is then left up to you to discern which one is best suited to your needs and requirements.

One specific diet clearly stands out above the rest, in terms of feasibility and nutritional soundness-and that is the Mediterranean diet. The Mediterranean sounds like a wonderful place to go on vacation, but do you know the answer when people ask you, what is Mediterranean diet?

Places of origin and various influences

As the name suggests, the diet owes its origins to the magnificent countries along the Mediterranean coast-Spain, Portugal, southern France, southern Italy, Greece, and areas in the Middle East.

The Mediterranean diet mainly consists of all types of fresh fruits and vegetables, nuts, legumes, unrefined cereals, whole grains, fish, seafood, eggs, poultry, healthy doses of olive oil and red wine, moderate servings of cheeses and yogurt, and occasional indulgences of red meat. Although the diet discourages the consumption of foods high in refined sugars and saturated fats, it does not ban entire food groups-and that makes it quite attractive for dieters of all ages and ethnicities.

Health aspects, safety, and efficiency in weight loss promotion

One of the health highlights of the Mediterranean diet is its heart-healthy q uality. Studies have shown that individuals who have adopted the diet into their lifestyles are at a lower risk for cardiovascular disease, among various other illnesses. This conclusion can be attributed to the diet's low amounts of saturated fat and abundance of health foods.

When coupled with an active lifestyle, the Mediterranean diet can guarantee maintainable weight loss. Such can easily be achieved, as the suggested foods will be able to provide the body with necessary fuel for sustainable energy throughout the day.

And because all types of foods can be eaten with the diet, all essential nutrients can be made available for the body's needs. Thus, the Mediterranean diet does not rob the body of any of its req uirements, and in other words, is completely safe.

Satisfaction in both fullness and taste

People who have embraced the Mediterranean diet do not view it as a typical diet, but as a healthier lifestyle choice. It is a choice that is considerably simple to stick to because it keeps you satiated for long periods of time, and taste is one of the many things that are not sacrificed.

The Mediterranean Diet is a healthy way of eating that was adopted by people who wanted to mimic the basic elements of the way that people in the Mediterranean countries eat. It follows the dietary patterns in such countries as Greece and Italy. But it is more than a diet. The Mediterranean Diet is a nutritional model.

So what is included in this diet? The most basic of Mediterranean diet recipes include things grown naturally from the earth: Fruits and vegetables, rice, cereals, and bread make up the basic components. Wheat is a staple in the Mediterranean Diet, as grain is imperative in any healthy diet. In this nutritional model, red wine and olive oil are also important staples. Different kinds of fish are as well.

Although this diet was introduced in the mid-1940s, it was not until the early 1990s that it really became noticed and began to pick up any speed. This is because people who live in that area of the world have been known to have significantly lower cholesterol levels. People who eat according to the various Mediterranean diet recipes also love it due to the fact that it has been rumored to have some cancer-fighting properties as well.

Is the Mediterranean Diet right for you? Is it time for you to jump on the bandwagon? Whether or not it's the right choice for you remains to be seen. It is, after all, just another way of eating. But there is certainly no denying that it is a much healthier way of eating. You can find green vegetables, calcium, and other important minerals and vitamins in the foods used in the preparation of many your more basic Mediterranean diet recipes.

So the next time someone asks you, what is Mediterranean diet, you can confidently say that it is a lifestyle choice that entails various benefits if adopted. History of the Mediterranean Diet

In recent years, a growing number of men and women in different countries around the world have become increasingly concerned about their health. Because of the fact that many people have become more concerned about their overall health, these men and women have paid closer attention to what they eat on a regular basis. In the final analysis, these men and women are making dietary decisions designed to improve their general health and wellbeing.

As people have become more conscious of their health and diet, a considerable number of these same men and women have become interested in the Mediterranean diet regimen. If you are, in fact, a person who appreciates the interrelationship between diet and health, you may have a definite interest in the history of the Mediterranean diet regimen.

Before you can appropriately understand what the Mediterranean diet is all about, you need to appreciate that it is more of a concept than a specific dining routine. In reality, there is no such thing as a Mediterranean diet common to all of the countries in the Mediterranean region of the world. Rather, the "Mediterranean diet" consists of those food items that people who live in the various nations in the region consume in common.

THE ORIGINS OF THE MEDITERRANEAN DIET

The concept of the Mediterranean diet is derived from the eating habits and patterns of the people who populate the countries of Italy, Greece, Spain, France, Tunisia, Lebanon and Morocco. As a result, the Mediterranean diet actually includes a tremendous array of delectable food. In point of fact, if a person elects to adopt the concept of the Mediterranean dining scheme, or if a person elects to follow a Mediterranean diet regimen, he or she will have the ability to enjoy a remarkable assortment of scrumptious fare.

The diet of the peoples that have populated the regions around the Mediterranean Sea actually have remained nearly completely unchanged for well over one thousand years. The history of the region is replete with examples of men and women living longer than similarly situated people who consumed alternate diets. Through the centuries, the people of the Mediterranean Sea region have enjoyed longer lives that people in other parts of the world at the same historical epoch.

At the heart of the Mediterranean diet are foods and beverages that are indigenous to the geographic landmass surrounding the Mediterranean Sea. In short, the development of the Mediterranean dieting and dining pattern initially developed by providence. The people of the region naturally and understandably ate those foods and drank those beverages that readily were available in and around their homes.

The Historical Elements of the Mediterranean Diet Scheme

As mentioned previously, over the centuries, the diet of the peoples of the Mediterranean Sea region has remained essentially unchanged. The Mediterranean diet consists of the bountiful consumption of a number of healthy food items including:

* Fresh fruit

* Fresh vegetables

* Low fat nuts

* Whole grains

* Monounsaturated fat

In a similar vein, the Mediterranean diet utilized by people for generation after generation excludes or limits certain food items that have been deemed harmful in recent scientific studies. These less than desirable food items include:

* Saturated fats

* Red and fatty meat

* Rich dairy products

* Fatty fish

The Historical Effects of the Mediterranean Diet Scheme

As has been alluded to earlier in this article on the history of the Mediterranean diet regimen, the people who inhabit the region have a demonstrably lower rate of heart disease and related ailments that oftentimes have a direct dietary connection. With the advent of scientific studies that have correlated the incidence of health problems with a poor diet, the positive effects of the Mediterranean diet have become self evident.

Research over the course of the past two decades has conclusively demonstrated that the men and women who populate the Mediterranean region are afflicted with heart disease and similar ailments far less often than people in other regions of the world. The experts who have conducted these studies have concluded that there is a strong likelihood that the diet scheme that is common in the Mediterranean region is responsible for maintaining the good health of the people who live in that corner of the globe throughout the past one thousand years.

During the past twenty years, a significant number of people in different countries around the world have turned their attention towards finding healthy diet regimens that are low in saturated fat and that include bountiful servings of fresh fruits and vegetable. Consequently, the Mediterranean diet has caught the eye of innumerable people who want to include healthy eating into their overall course of prudent living. In short, the Mediterranean diet encompasses foods and beverages that, when consumed in moderation, can work to lessen the threat of some serious diseases and can aid in creating the necessary foundation for a long, hearty lifetime.

THE MEDITERRANEAN DIET FOR LIFE

The Mediterranean "Diet" by nature is a very loose term and is applied by many with a wide array of interpretation. Whether it's location or geography, however, the Mediterranean region shares many common attributes regarding people, history, culture, climate, religion and certainly food.

Regardless of how you define the Mediterranean diet, it is still the best food to eat as far as health and fun are concerned. The Mediterranean diet, cuisine and lifestyle are the very things that have primarily shaped the people, their devotion to and love of the land which has built an undeniable passion for their way of life and cooking. The result is a worldwide appreciation for the Mediterranean cuisine as the ultimate for its tasty and healthy options.

A common misconception I've come across is that many people believe that the Mediterranean diet consists of a relatively small number of staple dishes. In fact, the beauty of the cuisine is that there are distinct differences as you go country to country in flavors, spices and other specialty ingredients as you go country to country...and yet, there remains a common string of characteristics throughout the region and individual countries. These are the essential elements of the Mediterranean diet, including food lower in saturated fats, high fiber content, a great emphasis on fruits, vegetables, legumes, grains, fresh herbs, lots of olive oil and an abundance of spices.

Make no mistake about it; one of the most crucial aspects of this diet is the overall lifestyle of the people living in the Mediterranean. The use of locally grown foods and fresh ingredients, the scarcity of red meat, and the geography all influence Mediterranean cuisine. Red meat is an occasional treat, especially around the holidays and special events. On the other hand, fish, poultry, eggs and cheese play a prominent role in the cuisine. Yet, this will vary in degree from the eastern part to the western part of the Mediterranean region. You will also see the differences in the consumption of wine, especially as dictated by societal and religious acceptance, tolerance or influence. Regardless of geography or climate there is an abundance of olive oil [the main fat], thus making it the main ingredient, influencing cooking style, life style, and providing an important link in the diversity and healthy aspect of the Mediterranean cuisine. During my childhood in Jordan and still to this day, olive oil remains the most important ingredient in all of Mediterranean cooking.

Many studies have been documented in support of the Mediterranean diet and the lifestyle and culture of the people that live in the region. Even with all the studies completed which have attributed good health to this diet; lifestyle also plays a large part in this determination. Let's not forget that physical activity and daily walking or exercise does go a long way in contributing to and reaping the benefits of such a diet.

So what exactly is the Mediterranean Diet? The following is the exact description which was delivered at a 1993 conference held at the Harvard School of Public Health: Plenty of fruit, vegetables, legumes, grains, with olive oil as the principle fat; lean red meat consumed only a few times per month and in small portions; moderate consumption of dairy products such as cheese, yogurt, fish, poultry and moderate consumption of wine at meal time.

The Staples of the Mediterranean Diet Include:

-Diligence about eating time and serving portions.

-Use of Olive Oil in all cooking and dressings.

-Use of whole grain, legumes and beans.

-Eating vegetables and fruit daily.

-Reducing the amount of saturated fats, especially the amount of red meat consumed.\

-Eating fish and nuts rich in omega-□3 fatty acids.

-Serving red wine with meals rather than other alcoholic drinks.

-Reducing the amount of salt in cooking and sugar, especially in buying packaged goods.

-Visiting your local farmers market more frequently.

-Choosing an exercise regimen consistent with your doctor's guidance.

-Eating Better, Fresher, Smarter overall and you will be happy you did!

Having grown up in the Mediterranean region and having lived and experienced the culture, I realize it is a way of life and way of thinking, and the respect for the land that enabled us to produce and grow the food we ate. Paying attention and being aware of what food is and where it comes from was considered sacred and a gift of the gods and was treated that way...we were not "above" food. It is with this attitude that food was treated whether it was raised or grown on the land we knew, owned and loved.

LOSING WEIGHT WITH THE MEDITERRANEAN DIET

The Mediterranean Diet has received a lot of media attention in recent years, owing to many celebrities' successes at losing weight on the diet. Based on the diets of people who live around the Mediterranean Sea, the diet places a high emphasis on being active, eating smaller portions, and enjoying the food you eat. Generally, eating red meat is kept to a minimum; protein sources of the diet include chicken, fish, cheese, and small amounts of eggs. Saturated fat is to be kept at a minimum.

The Mediterranean Diet is usually thought of as a "slow food" diet; emphasis is placed on cooking food at home rather than eating out at restaurants. Fast food is usually much too high in saturated fat to fit into the diet. With its emphasis on eating smaller amounts of healthy foods, the diet can help you lose weight quickly while still enjoying the food that you eat.

In addition to helping you lose weight, the diet also provides you with numerous health benefits. Olive oil and red wine are important parts of the Mediterranean Diet, and both are known to provide excellent health benefits. Olive oil is high in monounsaturated fats, which have been shown to raise levels of HDL cholesterol - the good form of cholesterol - and lower levels of LDL cholesterol - the bad cholesterol. Conversely, saturated fat has the opposite effect, and will greatly raise levels of LDL cholesterol.

Since the Mediterranean Diet is very low in saturated fat (the only real source being cheese) and very high in monounsaturated fat, it's considered very beneficial for heart health. Red wine is also beneficial for your cardiovascular system when consumed in moderate amounts, which is recommended by the diet. This is thought to be because of the high antioxidant content of grapes, which are also found in the wine produced from the grapes; antioxidants are known to protect your heart, your brain, and can prevent many types of cancer.

The diet places more emphasis on plant-based foods, such as whole grains and vegetables which contain large amounts of fiber. Fiber aids your digestive system and can help reduce your cholesterol levels, which also aids your cardiovascular health. Foods that are high in fiber are also usually quite low in calories while providing you with a feeling of fullness, which allows you to eat less calories while not going hungry, making the diet great for weight loss. Ultimately, the Mediterranean Diet is also a great choice for people who have a family history of heart disease, as it can greatly benefit your cardiovascular system.

The Mediterranean Diet is a healthy and sustainable diet that allows you to eat great-tasting food. It provides an emphasis on creating and enjoying the food that you eat, rather than mindlessly gorging yourself on fast food without regard to what you are eating. The diet helps to change your eating habits which leads to you successfully losing weight and keeping it off. There are many cookbooks available which have recipes tailored to the diet; you may find purchasing and using them useful.

REASONS WHY THE MEDITERRANEAN DIET IS A HEALTHY CHOICE IN THIS CENTURY

If you are a person who has been on the hunt for a solid diet plan, you may feel overwhelmed much of the time. In the 21st century it is nearly impossible for a person to turn on a television set or open a newspaper without being bombarded with advertisements for a variety of different diet plans and products.

With the tremendous array of diet plans, programs, supplements and aids on the market, it can seem nearly impossible to select a diet plan that can and will best meet your needs now and into the future. More importantly, it can be hard to discern if one or another of these various diet schemes actually is a healthy course to pursue. In many instances, fad diets really are not based on the fundamentals of healthy living.

As you go forward considering what type of diet plan or regimen will best serve your interests and improve your health into the future, you will want to take a look at the benefits that can be had through the Mediterranean diet.

While there are multiple reasons why the Mediterranean diet is a healthy approach, there are five primary reasons why the Mediterranean diet is a good choice.

1. The Benefits of Fruits, Vegetable, Fiber and Whole Grains

A major component of the Mediterranean diet includes the regular consumption of fresh fruits and vegetables. Medical experts and nutritionists universally agree that a person should eat between five and six servings of fresh fruits and vegetables (or steamed items) on a daily basis.

People who adhere to the Mediterranean diet actually end up eating more than the minimum recommended allowance of fruits and vegetables. As a result, nutritionists in different parts of the world have taken to recommending a Mediterranean based diet regimen to their clients. Similarly, doctors who consult with their patients about healthy eating practices oftentimes find themselves recommending the Mediterranean diet in this day and age.

Beyond fruits and vegetables, the Mediterranean diet includes healthy amounts of dietary fiber and whole grains. Fiber and whole grains have proven effective in lowering the incidence of heart disease and some types of cancer.

2. The Benefits of Olive Oil -- Avoiding Saturated Fat

Some people have a fundamental misperception about the Mediterranean diet. These people have heard that the Mediterranean diet is high in fat. On some level, there is some truth in the conception that the Mediterranean diet is higher in fat than are some other dieting programs. A person following the Mediterranean diet does take in about thirty percent of his or her daily calories from fat. (Most diets recommended the intake of calories from fat at the rate of about thirteen to fifteen percent per day. However, these diets are contemplating the ingesting of animal fat.)

The vast majority of fat that a person on the Mediterranean diet consumes comes from olive oil. In other words, the fat found in the Mediterranean diet is not the dangerous saturated fat that can cause disease, obesity and other health concerns. In fact, research has demonstrated that there are a number of solid benefits to consuming olive oil, including a reduction of the risk of the incidence of breast cancer in women.

3. Dairy in Moderation

While the consumption of low or non-fat dairy products in moderation can be beneficial in some instances, many people the world over rely on heavy creams, eggs and other fat filled dairy products in their daily diets. The Mediterranean diet is low in dairy. Indeed, any dairy products that actually are included within the diet regimen is low fat. A person is considered an extremely heavy egg eater if he or she consumes four eggs in a week.

4. Red Meat in Moderation

Very little red meat is included within the Mediterranean diet. When it comes to meat items, this diet relies on moderate amounts of lean poultry and fresh fish. As a result, people who follow the Mediterranean diet plan have lower levels of "bad" cholesterol and higher levels of "good: cholesterol.

In addition, because of the inclusion of lean, fresh fish in the diet, adherents to the Mediterranean diet enjoy the anti-oxidant benefits that are found in certain fish oils and products.

5. A Well Balanced Dieting Scheme

In the final analysis, the Mediterranean diet is gaining acclaim from experts and adherents the world over because it is a balanced dieting program. Study after study demonstrate that a balanced diet that is low in fat and that includes fruits, vegetable, whole grains and lean meat works to ensure total health and wellness.

The Mediterranean diet is a comprehensive regimen for healthy living. By following the strictures of the Mediterranean diet, a person can enjoy improved wellness, a reduction of the risk of certain diseases and, in many instances, a longer life.

15 BEST FOODS TO EAT FROM THE MEDITERRANEAN DIET

Could a Mediterranean diet be the diet to end all diets?

From Paleo to juicing to vegan, "diet" is not exactly a new word to the English language. But the food groups listed on the Mediterranean diet have us thinking this could be the ultimate answer if you're looking for a heart-healthy plan to shed the pounds and keep them off.

A Mediterranean diet is one that's rich in fruits, vegetables, nuts, fish, and whole grains, low in red meat, and free of refined foods and added sugars. More than just a diet, this is a way of living—by eating wholesome, good-for-you ingredients. There's no counting carbs or eating five times a day; you just have to stick to real food and forget all the artificially-made products out there. This diet has shown to improve the overall q uality of life, reduce the risk of chronic diseases, and also have a major connection with weight loss. To help you get on board, we've compiled your go-to grocery list for what to buy to get started. And for some helpful tips to purchasing these products on a budget, check out The 46 Best Supermarket Shopping Tips Ever!

EAT FREQUENTLY:

ALMONDS

Not only are they a natural way to help you lose weight, almonds also taste great as a snack, as milk, or as a nut butter. You can incorporate these power-packed nuts into a breakfast, lunch, or dinner dish, or even bring a handful for a snack. Research has shown that eating almonds prior to working out aids in dropping pounds q uicker; they're great to give you energy and super satiating. Nuts, in general, are high in protein but are a healthy fat—which means you should be eating them in moderation rather than mindlessly snacking. To make sure you don't go overboard on the almonds, pre-portion them by divvying up handful-size servings.

HUMMUS

Hummus can be a healthy dip or spread made simply by blending cooked garbanzo beans (chickpeas), tahini, olive oil, lemon juice, garlic, and spices of your choice. Chickpeas are loaded with protein and a surefire craving controller, so hummus is perfect for using as a dip with veggies like celery or cucumber. You can also make a variety of different hummus flavors like roasted red pepper, sundried tomato, or spicy jalapeno. It's also a fun way to give some livelihood to your sandwiches and pitas, too! There are plenty of hummus brands at the grocery store—but with such an easy recipe, we vote that you try making your own at home.

WILD SALMON

Ordering fish instead of a steak may seem like an effortless swap to help lighten the load, get in some added nutrients, and maybe even save room for that brownie (made using one of these 20 Best-Ever Tips and Swaps for Brownies). But what most don't know is that 99 percent of Atlantic salmon is being farm-raised and soy-fed, reaping nowhere close to the same benefits that wild salmon does. The farm-raised kind is packed with around 1,900 mg omega-6s— a fatty-acid that leads to inflammation. Instead, go to the local fish market and pick up the salmon that's specifically labeled as wild. Wild salmon has around 39 grams of protein per serving and a more reasonable amount of omega-6s, so the heart-healthy omega-3's aren't overwhelmed.

GARLIC

 Garlic is a great way to add some much-needed flavor to many dishes. From pasta to vegetables, there's no shortage of how far this little plant can take a meal. And it's not just for warding off the vampires; garlic also wards off bacteria, fungus, and body fat! It's filled with vitamins from manganese to vitamin B6 and super low in calories. Roast some garlic in the oven before combining it with cauliflower to create a soup like this one we love from Sweet Peas and Saffron.

EZEKIEL BREAD

Ezekiel bread is a sprouted ancient grain bread made with absolutely no sugar added. Instead of grabbing the white bread or the 'all-natural' whole grain bread (that's actually made with sugar and processed flours), go for Ezekiel bread. It comes in both classic sliced or tortilla wraps and packs in some extra flavor for your avocado toast or turkey sandwich. One slice has only 80 calories and a whopping 3 grams of fiber!

LEMON

Whether you're squeezing it into your water, tea, or over your chicken, lemon is a nutritional way to amp up your diet because you'll get a dose of vitamin C and waist-whiting detox benefits.

QUINOA

A vegetable quinoa soup is just one way to enjoy q uinoa. It can be used in energy bars, breakfast bowls, and even desserts. It's naturally gluten-free and a complete source of protein, with one cup cooked quinoa having around 8 grams of protein and 5 grams of fiber; this is a definite go-to for picking a grain. It's also low on the glycemic index and high in minerals like magnesium. Because it has a mild flavor, it's easy to make it sweet or savory by cooking it in things like coconut milk or chicken stock, with your choice of additions.

CAULIFLOWER

Of course the magical cauliflower is on the list of foods to freq uently dive into. This mighty vegetable is blasting with nutrients and minerals that are good for your health and easy to flavor. You can go the sweet or savory and turn this fibrous food into something fabulous! To get some the creativity flowing in the kitchen, check out these 17 Genius Ideas for Cooking With Cauliflower!

CHIA SEEDS

These little seeds have more power than appears. They are one of the best plant-based sources of omega-3s, with major anti-inflammatory properties and lessen the chances of heart disease. In just two tablespoons of chia seeds, you'll get 11 grams of fiber, which also keep you satisfied. Who knew such a small seed with such a big impact on your health? Try getting chia seeds into your diets by making a chia seed pudding or supercharging your breakfast smoothie. They're also great as a topping for oatmeals and yogurts to give it a little bite you need. They have almost no flavor so you won't be changing any taste—just adding tons of nutrients!

OLIVES & EVOO

There's a reason olive oil used to be a reward to the Olympians—it's valuable benefits are a gift to your health! Extra virgin olive oil has been cold-pressed from olives and it extremely useful in savory cooking. Filled with monounsaturated fats, EVOO is linked to helping reduce the risk of heart disease and may even help in fighting cancer. This kind of fat has also been seen to encourage weight loss by breaking down belly fat.

EAT MODERATELY:

EGGS

Eggs have an endless list of good-for-you health properties and can go with just about anything. And don't fall for the 'egg-whites only' option anymore. Research has proven that the taboo of eating the yolk is no longer because the yolk is actually the best part of the egg and its choline will aid weight loss. Make an omelet or bake up some egg muffins to grab on the go. You'll get a healthy dose of protein and get in some of that good cholesterol. And eggs aren't just for breakfast, check out these 10 Awesome Egg Dishes to Make For Dinner!

SKYR

Similar to Greek yogurt, skyr is Icelandic yogurt, but it has a thicker consistency and even more protein than Greek yogurt! This yogurt is strained an extra time and uses an extra cup of milk to get its great texture and bold flavor. Try Siggi's, which uses only natural ingredients like agave and fruit with milk from grass-fed cows and none of those artificial thickeners. Use a dollop on your soup or sprinkle in some of those chia seeds we talk so highly of. It's sure to make your belly happy, as well as your tastebuds. And to discover more types of yogurt, be sure to check out The 10 Types of Yogurt You Need to Know About.

CHICKEN

Whether grilled, baked or seared, chicken is an awesome protein to eat to fill you up without filling you out. Chicken has a light flavor on its own, but adding spices and seasonings means you can really make it your own masterpiece. Top a salad for lunch or make an entire dish by pairing it with a side of roasted veggies. To see how to get the most bang for your cluck, er, buck, check out 5 Rules For Buying The Healthiest Chicken!

EAT RARELY:

RED MEAT

We're not saying red meat should be totally exiled from the Mediterranean diet, but it shouldn't be your go-to staple. While it may be filled with protein—a good for you source of energy and weight loss aid—it also has a ton of iron. Yes, iron is good for you; but when too much iron is consumed, it actually increases the risk of weight gain and disease. Have no more than 6 ounces of red meat each week and stick to the grass-fed meats as often as possible for best results.

HEALTH BENEFITS OF MEDITERRANEAN DIET

The Mediterranean diet has many health benefits. Wondering researchers have spent years trying to discover why. Although many regions have adopted a much more westernized diet habit which has resulted in a mounting obesity issue, communities that still follow the traditional Mediterranean diet continue to experience health which is the envy of the western world.

The Mediterranean diet consists primarily of fresh, healthy plant food like whole grains, vegetables, fruits, nuts, legumes, olives, fish and seafood. They combine this with reduced amounts of red meat and dairy products.

The Mediterranean diet is more nutritious because foods are less processed. Processing food, and even cooking it, deprives it of nutrients. But in a traditional Mediterranean diet, most foods are eaten raw or lightly cooked. When red meat is served it is usually trimmed of excess fat. The overall diet provides plentiful fiber, healthy fats, vitamins, minerals, protein and essential fatty acids required by the body to maintain health and prevent chronic illnesses like heart disease and cancer.

Another notable aspect of the traditional Mediterranean diet is that not every meal contains animal flesh (i.e. meat or fish). There are commonly days with no animal flesh being consumed at all. On these days, the protein portion of the meal is derived from things like beans, nuts, seeds and eggs. Although eggs are still animal products, recent research indicates that eggs do NOT increase blood cholesterol as scientists and doctors used to believe. Another modern day alternative to meat is tofu which comes from soy beans. While this is not a part of the diet, it would certainly be a worthwhile addition to it.

All of these things result in the Mediterranean diet being high in monounsaturated fatty acids, otherwise known as M.U.F.As which are healthy fats. Diets containing M.U.F.As (and polyunsaturated fats, or P.U.F.As) rather than saturated and trans fats, tend to provide certain health benefits including reduced risk of:

- Heart disease
- High Cholesterol
- Stroke
- Cancer
- Type II Diabetes
- Parkinson's Disease
- Alzheimer's
- Depression
- Metabolic syndrome

Lets take a closer look at these.

Reduced risk of heart disease and high Cholesterol

High levels of saturated fats result in increased cholesterol in the bloodstream. Over time, the cholesterol attaches to the walls of arteries causing a narrowing of the arteries that can lead to blockages, heart attacks and heart disease. Quite clearly, the reduced amount of saturated fat in traditional Mediterranean diets results in lower cholesterol levels. In some cases, high cholesterol is hereditary and is caused by the liver producing too much. A healthy diet containing high amounts of Omega 3 fatty acids is proven to actively combat this issue and can have a significant lowering effect on cholesterol levels.

Reduced risk of Stroke

A Columbia University Medical Center study in which researchers followed 712 participants over a six year period discovered that participants who followed a moderate Mediterranean diet were 21% less likely to experience a stroke. Participants who followed a strict diet were 36% less likely to experience a stroke.

Reduced risk of cancer

According to a study by the Department of Clinical Sciences, University of Las Palmas de Gran Canaria, Spain: "There is a 'probable' protective role of the Mediterranean diet toward cancer in general." A National Cancer institute study of 500,000 people found that people who consumed more than 4 oz (113g) of red meat daily were 30% more likely to die from ANY cause over 10 years than those who consumed less. Sausages and processed meats increased the risk even more.

Reduced risk of Diabetes

Consumption of complex carbohydrates and high fiber foods reduces the Glycemic Index of foods and low GI foods prevent spikes in blood sugar levels. So a low GI diet such as the Mediterranean diet tends to prevent diabetes... See the section on Metabolic syndrome below

Reduced risk of Parkinson's & Alzheimer's

Some studies indicate that people who adhere to the Mediterranean diet have lower rates of Parkinson's and Alzheimer's diseases. Researchers are unsure why this is the case but they believe that healthy food choices improving cholesterol, blood sugar levels and blood vessel health may be the cause.

Reduced risk of Depression

British Researchers studied depression and diet in more than 3,000 middle-aged office workers for five years. Their findings indicated that people who ate a diet high in processed meat, chocolate, sugar, fried food, refined cereals and high-fat dairy products were more likely to suffer depression. But people who ate a diet rich in fruits, vegetables and fish similar to a Mediterranean diet were less likely to suffer depression. Their findings support other research that has found that healthy diets can protect against disease.

Reduced risk of Metabolic syndrome

Many overweight and obese people suffer from a condition called Metabolic Syndrome. Metabolic syndrome is a group of conditions - high blood pressure, a abnormal blood sugar levels, excessive body fat around the waist or abnormal cholesterol levels - that occur together. These increase the risk of heart disease, stroke and diabetes. People on the Mediterranean diet have been found to be less likely to be overweight, thus reducing incidence of this condition.

So, as you can see, adopting a traditional Mediterranean diet has many worthwhile health benefits. It has even been found to reverse many chronic diseases such as type II diabetes, high blood pressure, angina and even improving mobility in people who suffer from arthritis. So maybe it's time you tried this delicious, healthy diet!

10 REASONS WHY THE MEDITERRANEAN DIET IS GOOD FOR YOU

Low in Saturated Fat

Physicians and nutritionists the world over all agree that a diet that is high in saturated fat can have very negative consequences on a person's health and wellbeing. Indeed, a diet that is high in saturated fat can cause a person to suffer heart disease, can lead to cancer and can cause a whole host of other health problems and concern.

The Mediterranean diet is noteworthy because of the fact that it is very low in saturated fat. The typical person who follows the Mediterranean diet intakes less than eight percent of his or her calories from potentially harmful saturated fat. This is significantly below the average of people who do not follow a Mediterranean diet regimen.

Includes Plentiful Amounts of Fresh Fruits and Vegetables

Another reason why the Mediterranean diet is good for you lies in the fact that the diet includes the consumption of a significant amount of fruit and vegetables. Indeed, the diet encompasses more fresh fruits and vegetables than any other dietary program or plan today.

Fresh fruits and vegetables have a significant beneficial effect on a person's health and wellbeing. People who following the Mediterranean diet and consume generous servings of fruits and vegetables each day have a lower incidence of certain diseases including cancer and cardiovascular ailments.

High in Whole Grains and Fiber

A benefit in the Mediterranean diet is found in the fact that it lowers in the incidence of certain types of cancer. One of the reasons that the Mediterranean diet lowers the incidence of cancer is found in the fact that the diet is rich in whole grains and dietary fiber. Both whole grain and fiber have proven to lower the incidence of cancer, including colorectal cancer.

High in Anti-Oxidants

The Mediterranean diet is high in anti-oxidants. Anti-oxidants play a significant role in maintaining the body -- including organs, muscles and skin -- in top condition. A diet high in anti-oxidants is believed to ensure that a person will live a longer, healthier life.

Low in Red Meat

Because the Mediterranean diet is low in red meat, the diet plan works to reduce the amount of "bad cholesterol." A diet low in "bad cholesterol" lessens the incidence of cardiovascular disease, hypertension and stroke.

High in Lean Meats

The Mediterranean diet includes lean meats in moderate portions. The reasonable amount of lean meats -- including fish and certain seafood and fish -- provides a health source of protein and energy for a person.

Low in Dairy

The Mediterranean diet is low in dairy products. In fact, a true adherent to the Mediterranean diet includes almost no dairy products at all. Any dairy that is included in the diet is low fat or non fat. Because the diet is low in dairy, particularly fatty dairy products, the diet encourages a person to obtain or maintain an ideal weight. Additionally, the diet aids in reducing cholesterol and works to prevent heart disease.

Prevents Disease

As mentioned, one of the reasons that the Mediterranean diet is good for you rests in the fact that the diet plan appears to reduce the incidence of certain diseases including:

- Heart and cardiovascular disease
- Cancer
- Diabetes
- Hypertension
- Diabetes
- Longevity

The history of the people of the Mediterranean region demonstrates that the Mediterranean diet works to extend a person's life. In addition, while working to extend a person's life, this diet scheme works to ensure that a person's longer life will be healthy as well.

A Convenient Diet Program

Finally, the Mediterranean diet is good for you because it is a convenience diet program. In order to follow the Mediterranean diet you do not need to buy any special products or prepare a unique and hard to manage diet plan. If used with moderate exercise, it is a great way to lose weight while remaining healthy.

THE MEDITERRANEAN RECIPES DIET PLAN

The ingredients are fresh. The recipes are easy and perfect for those who find themselves with little time to prepare a healthy, tasty, and fresh meal for themselves and their families. It may take a little more time shopping, however, as none of the recipes use prepackaged ingredients with preservatives and fillers and all that other stuff with no nutritional value but lots of calories.

So just what is included in the Mediterranean Recipes diet? Most of the meals include bread (whole grain, of course), cheese, olive oil, fruits, nuts, grains, legumes, a variety of greens, and vegetables. Olive oil and lemon are two very important parts of Mediterranean cooking. Many spices such as oregano, basil, mint and type are widely used as is garlic. The food is simple but elegant with all different textures and flavors from very subtle to very robust. It is all very nutritious and healthy.

To begin this eating routine, there are a few things to keep in mind:

Your major sources of calcium should come from yogurt and good cheese. Salad dressings can be made from yogurt.

Red mean should only be consumed on rare occasion. It is fairy easy to use other ground meats such as turkey to make a burger eaten with some avocado and put on a whole wheat bun or pita.

You need to use seasonal and locally grown produce whenever possible to preserve the nutritional value of the food. Part of our lack of nutrients is due to the early picking of vegetable and fruit crops so they can be shipped around the world.

Make the recipes from scratch avoiding the use of pre-packaged ingredients. Again fresh is always better nutritionally and tastes better too.

Avoid sugary sweets and eat fruit, which is lower in calories and higher in fiber and nutrients.

Eat nuts such as almonds, walnuts, and cashews for a healthy, nutritious snack.

Protein sources are from lots of fish, some poultry and legumes. The omega-3 fatty acids in the fish will keep your heart and brain working at peak efficiency. Eggs are also a good source of protein.

All foods that need to be cooked should be baked or broiled and never fried.

Mediterranean Breakfast

Parmesan Spinach Cakes

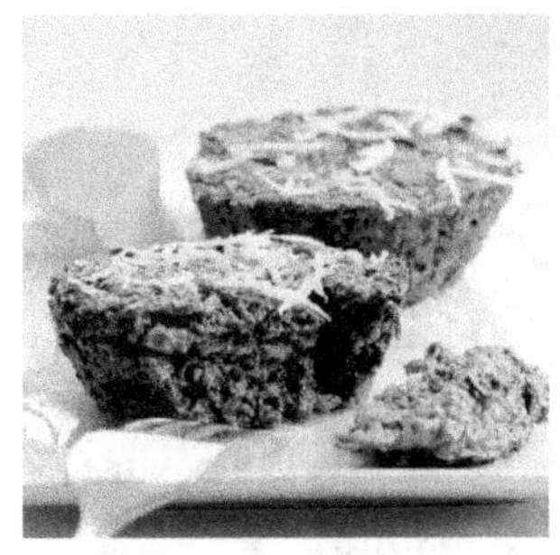

Ingredients 4 servings

12 ounces fresh spinach.

½ cup part-skim ricotta cheese, or low-fat cottage cheese

½ cup finely shredded Parmesan cheese, plus more for garnish

2 large eggs, beaten

1 clove garlic, minced

¼ teaspoon salt

¼ teaspoon freshly ground pepper

Preparation

Active 15 min

Ready In 40 min

Preheat oven to 400°F.

Pulse spinach in three batches in a food processor until finely chopped. Transfer to a medium bowl. Add ricotta (or cottage cheese), Parmesan, eggs, garlic, salt and pepper; stir to combine.

Coat 8 cups of the muffin pan with cooking spray. Divide the spinach mixture among the 8 cups (they will be very full).

Bake the spinach cakes until set, about 20 minutes. Let stand in the pan for 5 minutes. Loosen the edges with a knife and turn out onto a clean cutting board or large plate. Serve warm, sprinkled with more Parmesan, if desired.

Eq uipment: Muffin pan with 12 (½-cup) muffin cups

Note: Baby spinach is immature or young spinach—it's harvested earlier than large-leaved mature spinach. We like the sturdy texture of mature spinach in cooked dishes and serve tender, mild-flavored baby spinach raw or lightly wilted. Baby and mature spinach can be used interchangeably in these recipes (yields may vary slightly); be sure to remove the tough stems from mature spinach before using.

Weights & Measures 10 ounces trimmed mature spinach=about 10 cups raw 10 ounces baby spinach=about 8 cups raw

Nutrition information

Serving size: 2 spinach cakes

Per serving: 141 calories; 8 g fat(4 g sat); 2 g fiber; 6 g carbohydrates; 13 g protein; 182 mcg folate; 110 mg cholesterol; 1 g sugars; 0 g added sugars; 8,316 IU vitamin A; 24 mg vitamin C; 310 mg calcium; 3 mg iron; 448 mg sodium; 562 mg potassium

Wake-Up Smoothie

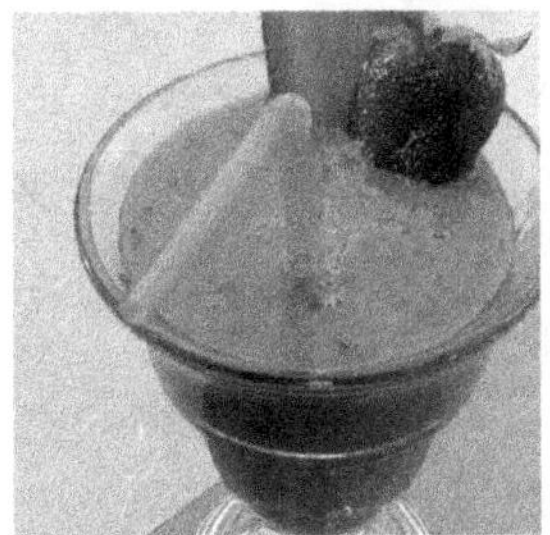

With a stash of berries in your freezer, you can jump-start your day with this nutritious, tasty smoothie in just minutes. It provides vitamin C, fiber, potassium and soy protein.

Ingredients 3 servings

1¼ cups orange juice, preferably calcium-fortified

1 banana

1¼ cups frozen berries, such as raspberries, blackberries, blueberries and/or strawberries

½ cup low-fat silken tofu, or low-fat plain yogurt

1 tablespoon sugar, or Splenda Granular (optional)

Preparation

Active

5 min

Ready In

5 min

Combine orange juice, banana, berries, tofu (or yogurt) and sugar (or Splenda), if using, in a blender; cover and blend until creamy. Serve immediately.

Nutrition information

Serving size: 1 cup

Per serving: 139 calories; 2 g fat(0 g sat); 4 g fiber; 28 g carbohydrates; 4 g protein; 50 mcg folate; 0 mg cholesterol; 17 g sugars; 0 g added sugars; 264 IU vitamin A; 66 mg vitamin C; 25 mg calcium; 1 mg iron; 19 mg sodium; 421 mg potassium

Breakfast Blueberry-Oatmeal Cakes

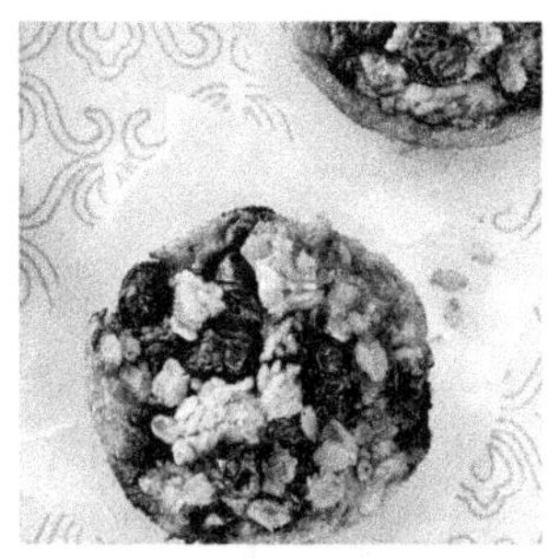

This oatmeal-meets-muffin-tin cake recipe is perfect for having a healthy breakfast available on busy weekdays. Make a batch on the weekend and keep them in your freezer. For a grab-and-go breakfast, reheat the oatmeal cakes in the microwave for about 40 seconds.

Ingredients 6 servings

2½ cups old-fashioned rolled oats

1½ cups low-fat milk

1 large egg, lightly beaten

¾ cup pure maple syrup

2 tablespoons canola oil

1 teaspoon vanilla extract

1 teaspoon ground cinnamon

1 teaspoon baking powder

¼ teaspoon salt

¾ cup blueberries, fresh or frozen

Preparation

Active

15 min

Ready In

55 min

Combine oats and milk in a large bowl. Cover and let soak in the refrigerator until much of the liq uid is absorbed, at least 8 hours and up to 12 hours.

Preheat oven to 375°F. Coat a 12-cup nonstick muffin tin with cooking spray.

Stir egg, maple syrup, oil, vanilla, cinnamon, baking powder and salt into the soaked oats until well combined. Divide the mixture among the muffin cups (about ¼ cup each). Top each with 1 tablespoon blueberries.

Bake the oatmeal cakes until they spring back when touched, 25 to 30 minutes. Let cool in the pan for 10 minutes. Loosen and remove with a paring knife. Serve warm.

Make Ahead Tip: Wrap airtight and refrigerate for up to 2 days or freeze for up to 3 months.

Eq uipment: Nonstick muffin tin with 12 (½-cup) cups

Storage smarts: For long-term freezer storage, wrap your food in a layer of plastic wrap followed by a layer of foil. The plastic will help prevent freezer burn while the foil will help keep off-odors from seeping into the food.

People with celiac disease or gluten-sensitivity should use oats that are labeled "gluten-free," as oats are often cross-contaminated with wheat and barley.

Nutrition information

Serving size: 2 oatmeal cakes

Per serving: 264 calories; 9 g fat(1 g sat); 4 g fiber; 41 g carbohydrates; 7 g protein; 24 mcg folate; 34 mg cholesterol; 17 g sugars; 12 g added sugars; 176 IU vitamin A; 2 mg vitamin C; 150 mg calcium; 2 mg iron; 219 mg sodium; 277 mg potassium

Oatmeal-Rhubarb Porridge

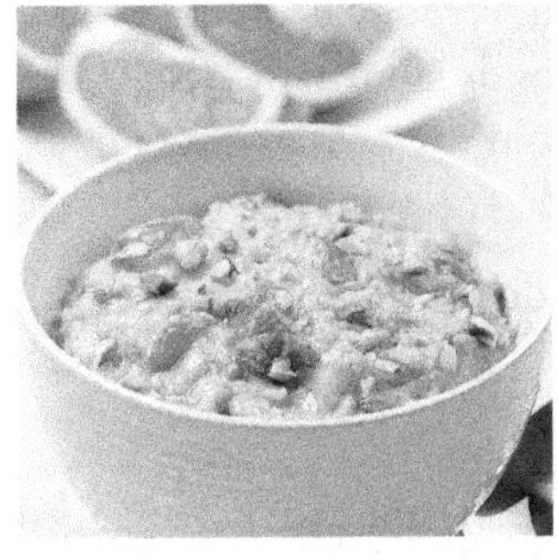

Perk up your morning oatmeal with the addition of tangy rhubarb. Using milk for this oatmeal gives it a calcium boost, but the recipe also works well with water—and you'll save about 60 calories.

Ingredients 2 servings

1½ cups nonfat milk or nondairy milk, such as soymilk or almond milk

½ cup orange juice

1 cup old-fashioned rolled oats

1 cup ½-inch pieces rhubarb, fresh or frozen

½ teaspoon ground cinnamon

Pinch of salt

2-3 tablespoons brown sugar, pure maple syrup or agave syrup

2 tablespoons chopped pecans or other nuts, toasted (see Tip) if desired

Preparation

Active

20 min

Ready In

20 min

Combine milk, juice, oats, rhubarb, cinnamon and salt in a medium saucepan. Bring to a boil over medium-high heat. Reduce heat, cover and cook at a very gentle bubble, stirring freq uently, until the oats and rhubarb are tender, about 5 minutes. Remove from the heat and let stand, covered, for 5 minutes. Stir in sweetener to taste. Top with nuts.

Tip: To toast chopped nuts, place in a small dry skillet and cook over medium-low heat, stirring constantly, until fragrant and lightly browned, 2 to 4 minutes.

People with celiac disease or gluten-sensitivity should use oats that are labeled "gluten-free," as oats are often cross-contaminated with wheat and barley.

Nutrition information

Serving size: 1 generous cup

Per serving: 336 calories; 8 g fat(1 g sat); 6 g fiber; 56 g carbohydrates; 13 g protein; 53 mcg folate; 4 mg cholesterol; 25 g sugars; 9 g added sugars; 567 IU vitamin A; 36 mg vitamin C; 302 mg calcium; 2 mg iron; 153 mg sodium; 772 mg potassium

Muffin-Tin Quiches with Smoked Cheddar & Potato

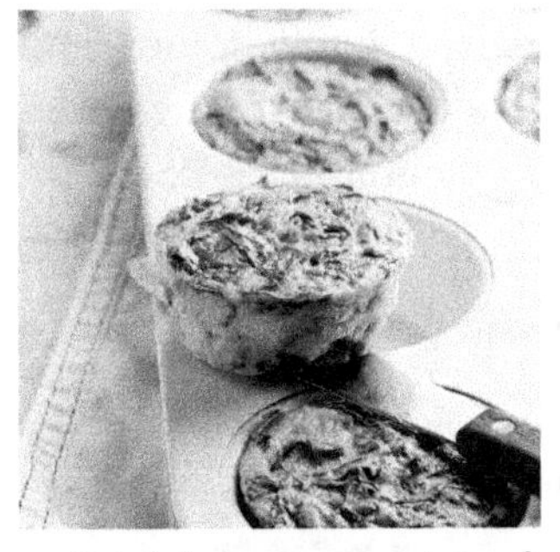

Potatoes, cheese and greens make this mini q uiche recipe delicious and satisfying. Bake up a batch over the weekend and you'll have breakfast available in a hurry for the rest of the week.

Ingredients 6 servings

2 tablespoons extra-virgin olive oil

1½ cups finely diced red-skinned potatoes

1 cup diced red onion

¾ teaspoon salt, divided

8 large eggs

1 cup shredded smoked Cheddar cheese

½ cup low-fat milk

½ teaspoon ground black pepper

1½ cups chopped fresh spinach

Preparation

Prep

30 min

Ready In

1 h

Preheat oven to 325°F. Coat a 12-cup muffin tin with cooking spray.

Heat oil in a large skillet over medium heat. Add potatoes, onion and ¼ teaspoon salt and cook, stirring, until the potatoes are just cooked through, about 5 minutes. Remove from heat and let cool 5 minutes.

Whisk eggs, cheese, milk, pepper and the remaining ½ teaspoon salt in a large bowl. Stir in spinach and the potato mixture. Divide the q uiche mixture among the prepared muffin cups.

Bake until firm to the touch, about 25 minutes. Let stand 5 minutes before removing from the tin.

Nutrition information

Serving size: 2 q uiches each

Per serving: 238 calories; 16 g fat(5 g sat); 1 g fiber; 11 g carbohydrates; 14 g protein; 59 mcg folate; 263 mg cholesterol; 3 g sugars; 0 g added sugars; 1,251 IU vitamin A; 7 mg vitamin C; 177 mg calcium; 2 mg iron; 494 mg sodium; 377 mg potassium

Egg & Salmon Sandwich

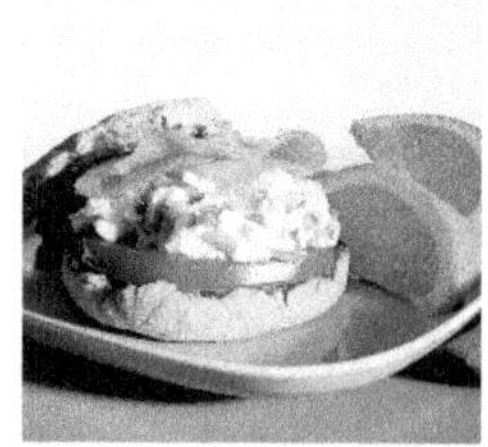

Smoked salmon and egg whites on a toasted whole-wheat English muffin is the perfect power breakfast. For a more substantial meal, pair it with a piece of fruit or a glass of 100% juice.

Ingredients 1 serving

½ teaspoon extra-virgin olive oil

1 tablespoon finely chopped red onion

Onions Red

2 large egg whites, beaten

Pinch of salt

½ teaspoon capers, rinsed and chopped (optional)

1 ounce smoked salmon

1 slice tomato

1 whole-wheat English muffin, split and toasted

Preparation

Active

15 min

Ready In

15 min

Heat oil in a small nonstick skillet over medium heat. Add onion and cook, stirring, until it begins to soften, about 1 minute. Add egg whites, salt and capers (if using) and cook, stirring constantly, until whites are set, about 30 seconds.

To make the sandwich, layer the egg whites, smoked salmon and tomato on English muffin.

Nutrition information

Serving size: 1 sandwich

Per serving: 230 calories; 5 g fat(1 g sat); 5 g fiber; 29 g carbohydrates; 18 g protein; 40 mcg folate; 7 mg cholesterol; 7 g sugars; 2 g added sugars;

195 IU vitamin A; 3 mg vitamin C; 187 mg calcium; 2 mg iron; 687 mg sodium; 358 mg potassium

Mexi-Melt

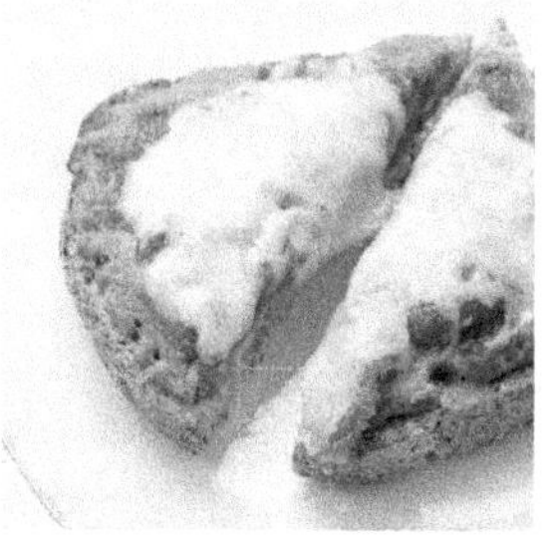

Spread leftover refried beans on whole-wheat toast and top with salsa and cheese for an easy breakfast that has plenty of staying power.

Ingredients 1 serving

2 tablespoons canned nonfat refried beans

1 slice whole-wheat bread, toasted

Organics Mild Salsa Organic

1 tablespoon prepared salsa

1 tablespoon shredded cheese, such as Mexican blend or Jack

Preparation

Active

10 m

Ready In

10 m

Spread beans on toast. Top with salsa, then cheese. Microwave on High until the cheese is melted and the beans are hot, about 45 seconds.

Nutrition information

Per serving: 124 calories; 3 g fat(2 g sat); 3 g fiber; 17 g carbohydrates; 7 g protein; 30 mcg folate; 6 mg cholesterol; 2 g sugars; 1 g added sugars; 132 IU vitamin A; 1 mg vitamin C; 112 mg calcium; 1 mg iron; 409 mg sodium; 222 mg potassium

Quick Breakfast Taco

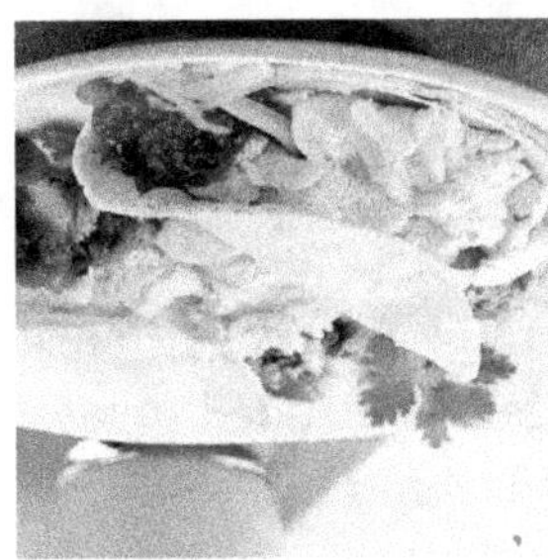

A smaller cousin of the breakfast burrito, the breakfast taco made with reduced-fat Cheddar and egg substitute is a satisfying and healthy breakfast option.

Ingredients 1 serving

2 corn tortillas

1 tablespoon salsa

2 tablespoons shredded reduced-fat Cheddar cheese

½ cup liquid egg substitute, such as Egg Beaters

Egg Beaters Product Regular

Preparation

Active

15 m

Ready In

15 m

Top tortillas with salsa and cheese. Heat in the microwave until the cheese is melted, about 30 seconds.

Meanwhile coat a small nonstick skillet with cooking spray. Heat over medium heat, add egg substitute and cook, stirring, until the eggs are cooked through, about 90 seconds. Divide the scrambled egg between the tacos.

Nutrition information

Serving size: 2 tacos

Per serving: 239 calories; 7 g fat(2 g sat); 3 g fiber; 24 g carbohydrates; 21 g protein; 23 mcg folate; 4 mg cholesterol; 2 g sugars; 0 g added sugars; 559 IU vitamin A; 0 mg vitamin C; 169 mg calcium; 3 mg iron; 480 mg sodium; 558 mg potassium

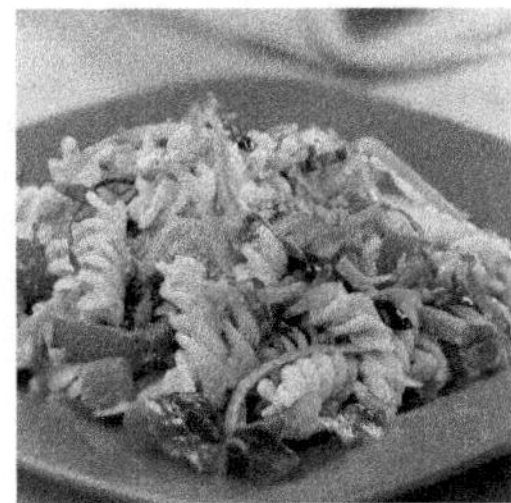

Mediterranean Lunch

Garden Pasta Salad

This lightly dressed pasta salad gets lots of flavor from kalamata olives and basil. A colorful mix of diced bell pepper, shredded carrot and tomatoes adds vitamins and minerals. Serve on a crisp bed of greens. Toss in canned chunk light tuna, cooked chicken or flavored baked tofu to add protein and make it more substantial.

Ingredients 6 servings

2 cups whole-wheat rotini, (6 ounces)

¾ cup reduced-fat mayonnaise

¾ cup low-fat plain yogurt

2 tablespoons extra-virgin olive oil

1 tablespoon red-wine vinegar, or lemon juice

1 clove garlic, minced

¾teaspoon salt

1 cup cherry or grape tomatoes, halved

Freshly ground pepper, to taste

1 cup diced yellow or red bell pepper, (1 small)

1 cup grated carrots, (2-4 carrots)

½ cup chopped pitted kalamata olives

½ cup chopped scallions, (4 scallions)

¾ cup slivered fresh basil

Preparation

Active

35 min

Ready In

35 min

Bring a large pot of lightly salted water to a boil. Cook pasta, stirring occasionally, until just tender, 8 to 10 minutes, or according to package directions. Drain and refresh under cold running water.

Whisk mayonnaise, yogurt, oil, vinegar (or lemon juice), garlic, salt and pepper in a large bowl until smooth. Add the pasta and toss to coat. Add tomatoes, bell pepper, carrots, scallions, olives and basil; toss to coat well.

Nutrition information

Serving size: 1 cup

Per serving: 217 calories; 9 g fat(1 g sat); 4 g fiber; 30 g carbohydrates; 6 g protein; 32 mcg folate; 4 mg cholesterol; 5 g sugars; 1 g added sugars; 4,338 IU vitamin A; 39 mg vitamin C; 70 mg calcium; 2 mg iron; 267 mg sodium; 272 mg potassium

Mediterranean Tuna Antipasto Salad

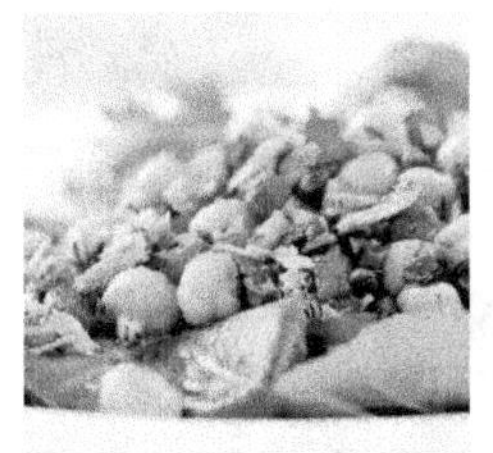

Packed with protein and fiber, this tuna and bean salad is ready in a flash. For an extra kick, add a pinch of crushed red pepper or cayenne.

Ingredients 4 servings

1 15- to 19-ounce can beans, such as chickpeas, black-eyed peas or kidney beans, rinsed

2 5- to 6-ounce cans water-packed chunk light tuna, drained and flaked

1 large red bell pepper, finely diced

½ cup finely chopped red onion

½ cup chopped fresh parsley, divided

4 teaspoons capers, rinsed

1½ teaspoons finely chopped fresh rosemary

½ cup lemon juice, divided

4 tablespoons extra-virgin olive oil, divided

Freshly ground pepper, to taste

¼ teaspoon salt

8 cups mixed salad greens

Preparation

Active

25 min

Ready In

25 min

Combine beans, tuna, bell pepper, onion, parsley, capers, rosemary, ¼ cup lemon juice and 2 tablespoons oil in a medium bowl. Season with pepper. Combine the remaining ¼ cup lemon juice, 2 tablespoons oil and salt in a large bowl. Add salad greens; toss to coat. Divide the greens among 4 plates. Top each with the tuna salad.

Note: Chunk light tuna, which comes from the smaller skipjack or yellowfin, has less mercury than canned white albacore tuna. The FDA/EPA advises that women who are or might become pregnant, nursing mothers and young children consume no more than 6 ounces of albacore a week; up to 12 ounces of canned light tuna is considered safe.

Nutrition information

Per serving: 306 calories; 16 g fat(2 g sat); 8 g fiber; 28 g carbohydrates; 15 g protein; 223 mcg folate; 15 mg cholesterol; 4 g sugars; 0 g added sugars; 4,961 IU vitamin A; 97 mg vitamin C; 115 mg calcium; 4 mg iron; 467 mg sodium; 752 mg potassium

Turkey & Tomato Panini

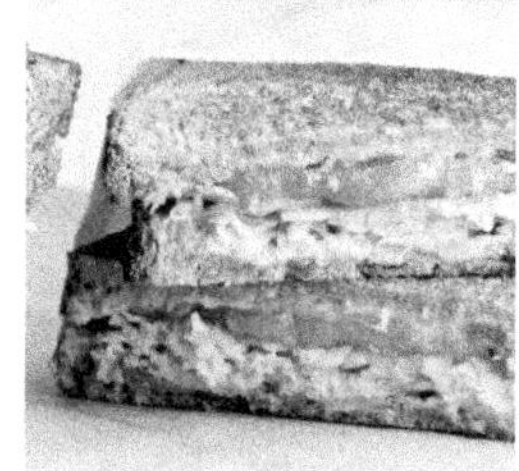

A creamy spread full of Parmesan and fresh basil cozies up to turkey and summer-ripe tomato slices for a savory hot sandwich that will q uickly become a go-to mealtime solution.

Ingredients 4 servings

3 tablespoons reduced-fat mayonnaise

2 tablespoons nonfat plain yogurt

2 tablespoons shredded Parmesan cheese

2 tablespoons chopped fresh basil

1 teaspoon lemon juice

Freshly ground pepper, to taste

8 ounces thinly sliced reduced-sodium deli turkey

8 tomato slices

8 slices whole-wheat bread

2 teaspoons canola oil

Preparation

Active

25 min

Ready In

25 min

Have four 15-ounce cans and a medium skillet (not nonstick) ready by the stove.

Combine mayonnaise, yogurt, Parmesan, basil, lemon juice and pepper in a small bowl. Spread about 2 teaspoons of the mixture on each slice of bread. Divide turkey and tomato slices among 4 slices of bread; top with the remaining bread.

Heat 1 teaspoon canola oil in a large nonstick skillet over medium heat. Place 2 panini in the pan. Place the medium skillet on top of the panini, then weigh it down with the cans. Cook the panini until golden on one side, about 2 minutes. Reduce the heat to medium-low, flip the panini, replace the top skillet and cans, and cook until the second side is golden,

1 to 3 minutes more. Repeat with another 1 teaspoon oil and the remaining panini.

Nutrition information

Per serving: 314 calories; 8 g fat(1 g sat); 5 g fiber; 37 g carbohydrates; 22 g protein; 10 mcg folate; 30 mg cholesterol; 6 g sugars; 495 IU vitamin A; 7 mg vitamin C; 135 mg calcium; 3 mg iron; 715 mg sodium; 139 mg potassium

Tuscan-Style Tuna Salad

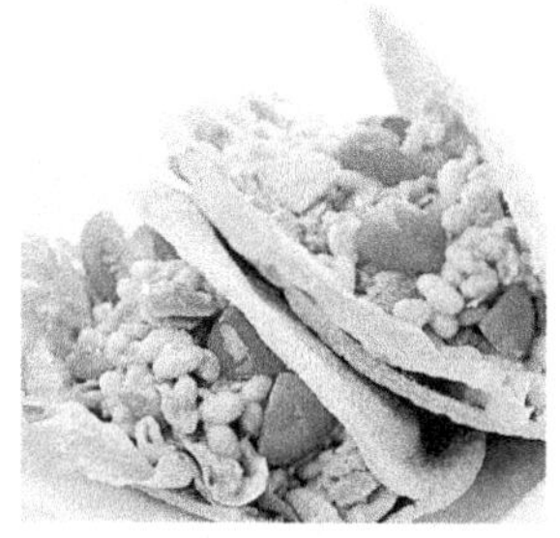

This streamlined version of a northern Italian idea is perfect for a summer evening: no-fuss, no-cook and big taste. You can even make it ahead and store it, covered, in the refrigerator for several days. If you do, use it as a wrap filling for the next day's lunch.

Ingredients 4 servings

2 6-ounce cans chunk light tuna, drained

10 cherry tomatoes, q uartered

4 scallions, trimmed and sliced

2 tablespoons extra-virgin olive oil

2 tablespoons lemon juice

¼ teaspoon salt

1 15-ounce can small white beans, such as cannellini or great northern, rinsed (see Ingredient note)

Freshly ground pepper, to taste

Preparation

Active

10 min

Ready In

10 min

Combine tuna, beans, tomatoes, scallions, oil, lemon juice, salt and pepper in a medium bowl. Stir gently. Refrigerate until ready to serve.

Make Ahead Tip: Cover and refrigerate for up to 2 days.

Notes: Chunk light tuna, which comes from the smaller skipjack or yellowfin, has less mercury than canned white albacore tuna. The FDA/EPA advises that women who are or might become pregnant, nursing mothers and young children consume no more than 6 ounces of albacore a week; up to 12 ounces of canned light tuna is considered safe.

When you use canned beans in a recipe, be sure to rinse them first in a colander under cold running water, as their canning liquid often contains a fair amount of sodium.

Nutrition information

Serving size: 1 cup

Per serving: 199 calories; 9 g fat(1 g sat); 6 g fiber; 20 g carbohydrates; 16 g protein; 102 mcg folate; 17 mg cholesterol; 2 g sugars; 0 g added sugars; 488 IU vitamin A; 11 mg vitamin C; 73 mg calcium; 2 mg iron; 555 mg sodium; 549 mg potassium

Ravioli & Vegetable Soup

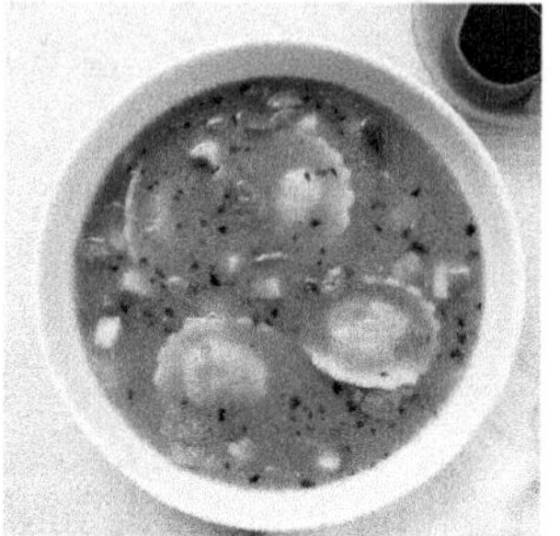

Fresh or frozen ravioli cook in minutes and turn this light vegetable soup into a main course. Look for whole-wheat or whole-grain ravioli in the refrigerated or frozen section of the supermarket. Tortellini can be used instead of ravioli as well.

Ingredients 4 servings

1 tablespoon extra-virgin olive oil

Pompeian Olive Oil Extra Virgin

2 cups frozen bell pepper and onion mix, thawed and diced

2 cloves garlic, minced

¼ teaspoon crushed red pepper, or to taste (optional)

1 28-ounce can crushed tomatoes, preferably fire-roasted

1 15-ounce can vegetable broth or reduced-sodium chicken broth

1½ cups hot water

1 teaspoon dried basil or marjoram

1 6- to 9-ounce package fresh or frozen cheese (or meat) ravioli, preferably whole-wheat

2 cups diced zucchini, (about 2 medium)

Freshly ground pepper to taste

Preparation

Active

25 min

Ready In

25 min

Heat oil in a large saucepan or Dutch oven over medium heat. Add pepper-onion mix, garlic and crushed red pepper (if using) and cook, stirring, for 1 minute. Add tomatoes, broth, water and basil (or marjoram); bring to a rolling boil over high heat. Add ravioli and cook for 3 minutes less than the package directions. Add zucchini; return to a boil. Cook until the zucchini is crisp-tender, about 3 minutes. Season with pepper.

Make Ahead Tip: Cover and refrigerate for up to 3 days. Thin with broth before reheating, if desired.

Nutrition information

Serving size: about 2 cups

Per serving: 261 calories; 8 g fat(3 g sat); 7 g fiber; 33 g carbohydrates; 11 g protein; 16 mcg folate; 28 mg cholesterol; 12 g sugars; 0 g added sugars; 2,279 IU vitamin A; 24 mg vitamin C; 97 mg calcium; 5 mg iron; 354 mg sodium; 732 mg potassium

Mediterranean Wrap

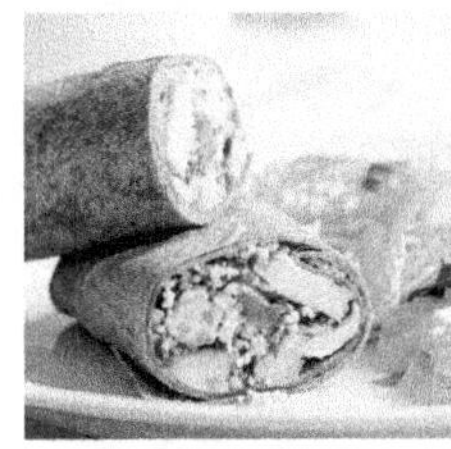

This wrap is stuffed with chicken tenders and couscous with a hit of lemon and a healthy dose of fresh herbs. Save any leftovers to wrap up for an easy lunch. Serve with: Mixed green salad and a glass of crisp white wine.

Ingredients 4 servings

½ cup water

½ cup couscous, preferably whole-wheat

1 cup chopped fresh parsley

½ cup chopped fresh mint

¼ cup lemon juice

3 tablespoons extra-virgin olive oil

2 teaspoons minced garlic

¼ teaspoon salt, divided

¼ teaspoon freshly ground pepper

1 pound chicken tenders

1 medium tomato, chopped

Tomatoes On the Vine

1 cup chopped cucumber

4 10-inch spinach or sun-dried tomato wraps or tortillas

Preparation

Active

40 min

Ready In

40 min

Bring water to a boil in a small saucepan. Stir in couscous and remove from the heat. Cover and let stand for 5 minutes. Fluff with a fork. Set aside.

Meanwhile, combine parsley, mint, lemon juice, oil, garlic, ? teaspoon salt and pepper in a small bowl.

Toss chicken tenders in a medium bowl with 1 tablespoon of the parsley mixture and the remaining ? teaspoon salt. Place the tenders in a large nonstick skillet and cook over medium heat until cooked though, 3 to 5 minutes per side. Transfer to a clean cutting board. Cut into bite-size pieces when cool enough to handle.

Stir the remaining parsley mixture into the couscous along with tomato and cucumber.

To assemble wraps, spread about ¾ cup of the couscous mixture onto each wrap. Divide the chicken among the wraps. Roll the wraps up like a burrito, tucking in the sides to hold the ingredients in. Serve cut in half.

Eat neat: Keeping the filling inside a wrap or burrito can be a challenge, especially if you're on the go. That's why we recommend wrapping your burrito in foil so you can pick it up and eat it without losing the filling, peeling back the foil as you go.

Nutrition information

Serving size: 1 wrap

Per serving: 510 calories; 18 g fat(3 g sat); 6 g fiber; 55 g carbohydrates; 32 g protein; 192 mcg folate; 63 mg cholesterol; 5 g sugars; 0 g added sugars; 2,027 IU vitamin A; 33 mg vitamin C; 165 mg calcium; 6 mg iron; 726 mg sodium; 564 mg potassium

Mediterranean Dessert

Greek Iced Coffee

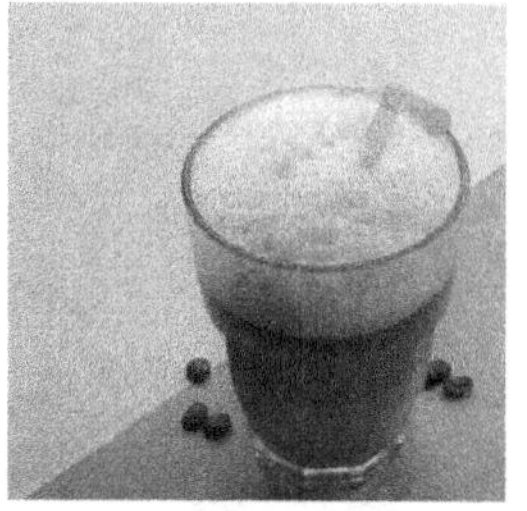

This frothy delight is a great summer treat when the summer heat makes hot coffee less appealing.

Ingredients 1 serving

  2 teaspoons instant coffee

  1-2 teaspoons sugar

2 ice cubes

¼ cup cold water

1 cup chilled milk

Preparation

  Active

  5 m

  Ready In

  15 m

Place instant coffee, sugar, ice cubes and water in a jar with a tight-fitting lid; shake vigorously for 30 seconds, or until frothy. Stir in milk.

Nutrition information

  Serving size: ½ cup

  Per serving: 57 calories; 1 g fat(1 g sat); 0 g fiber; 10 g carbohydrates; 3 g protein; 4 mcg folate; 4 mg cholesterol; 8 g sugars; 4 g added sugars;

159 IU vitamin A; 0 mg vitamin C; 106 mg calcium; 0 mg iron; 38 mg sodium; 193 mg potassium

Double Peanut Butter-Chocolate Chewies

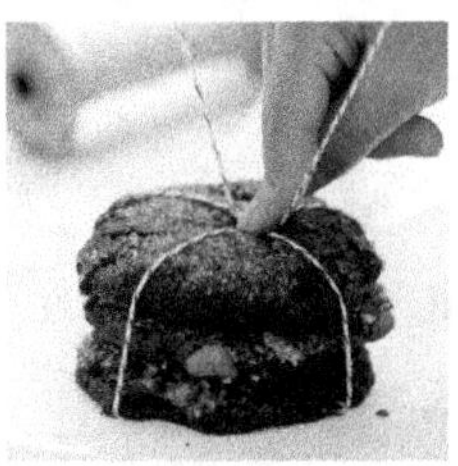

These soft chocolate cookies have a big peanut flavor since they use peanut butter and peanut butter chips.

ingredient

1 cup chunky natural peanut butter

¼ cup canola oil

½ cup packed dark brown sugar

½ cup granulated sugar

2 large eggs

3 tablespoons low-fat plain yogurt

1 tablespoon vanilla extract

¾ cup all-purpose flour

¾ cup of unsweetened cocoa powder

¼ cup rolled oats

1 teaspoon baking soda

½ teaspoon salt

¼ cup semisweet chocolate chips

¼ cup trans-fat-free peanut butter chips, such as Sunspire

¼ cup turbinado sugar (see Note)

Preparation

Active

1 h

Ready In

1 h 30 m

Preheat oven to 350°F.

Beat peanut butter, oil, brown sugar and granulated sugar in a large bowl with an electric mixer on medium speed until the sugars are blended. Beat in eggs, yogurt and vanilla until combined.

Whisk flour, cocoa, oats, baking soda and salt in a medium bowl. With the mixer on low speed, gradually add the dry ingredients to the peanut butter mixture until blended. (It will be sticky.) Stir in chocolate and peanut butter chips.

Using a small cookie scoop or slightly rounded tablespoons of dough, place cookies 2 inches apart on ungreased cookie sheets.

Dip the bottom of a glass in water and then in turbinado sugar. Use the sugared glass to flatten the cookies slightly, leaving a thin layer of sugar on top, rewetting the glass as needed.

Bake the cookies in batches until they are just set and the tops appear cracked, 8 to 10 minutes. (Do not overbake or they will be dry.) Cool on the baking sheet for 2 minutes before transferring to a wire rack to cool.

Make Ahead Tip: Store in an airtight container for up to 3 days or freeze for up to 3 months.

Ingredient Note: Turbinado sugar is steam-cleaned raw cane sugar. It's coarse-grained and light brown in color, with a slight molasses flavor. Find it in the natural-foods section of large supermarkets or at natural-foods stores.

Storage smarts: To extend the life of your baked goods, store them in an airtight container in a single layer or between layers of parchment paper to prevent sticking.

Nutrition information

Serving size: 1 cookie

Per serving: 117 calories; 6 g fat(1 g sat); 1 g fiber; 13 g carbohydrates; 3 g protein; 10 mcg folate; 10 mg cholesterol; 9 g sugars; 8 g added sugars; 16 IU vitamin A; 0 mg vitamin C; 8 mg calcium; 0 mg iron; 95 mg sodium; 33 mg potassium

Yummy Molasses Crackles

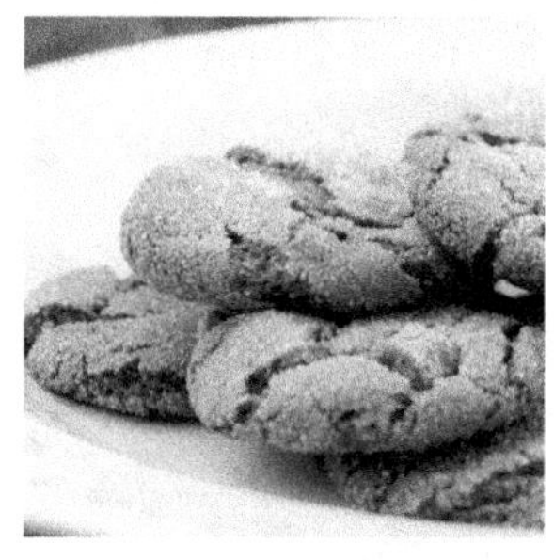

Ingredients 36 servings

 ¼ cup unsalted butter, softened

 1 cup plus? Cup sugar, divided

 1 large egg, beaten

 ¼ cup molasses

2 cups all-purpose flour

2 teaspoons baking soda

1 teaspoon ground cinnamon

½ teaspoon salt

¼ teaspoon ground cloves

⅔ Teaspoon ground ginger

⅔ Cup crystallized ginger, finely chopped

Preparation

Active

15 m

Ready In

1 h 30 m

Beat butter and 1 cup sugar in a large bowl with an electric mixer until creamy. Add egg and molasses. Mix well.

Whisk flour, baking soda, cinnamon, salt, cloves and ginger in another large bowl until well blended. Stir in crystallized ginger.

Blend the flour mixture into the butter mixture a cup at a time, mixing well, until it is all incorporated. Chill the dough in the refrigerator until firm, 30 minutes to 1 hour.

Preheat oven to 375°F. Lightly coat 2 baking sheets with cooking spray.

Place the remaining ? cup sugar in a shallow dish. Roll the dough into 1-inch balls and then roll in the sugar. Place 1½ inches apart on the prepared baking sheet.

Bake the cookies, in batches, until they crackle on top, 8 to 10 minutes. Transfer to a wire rack to cool.

Make Ahead Tip: Store in an airtight container at room temperature for up to 5 days or freeze for up to 3 months.

Storage smarts: To extend the life of your baked goods, store them in an airtight container in a single layer or between layers of parchment paper to prevent sticking.

Nutrition information

Serving size: 1 cookie

Per serving: 79 calories; 1 g fat(1 g sat); 0 g fiber; 16 g carbohydrates; 1 g protein; 21 mcg folate; 9 mg cholesterol; 10 g sugars; 9 g added sugars; 74 IU vitamin A; 0 mg vitamin C; 10 mg calcium; 1 mg iron; 106 mg sodium; 43 mg potassium

One-Bowl Chocolate Cake

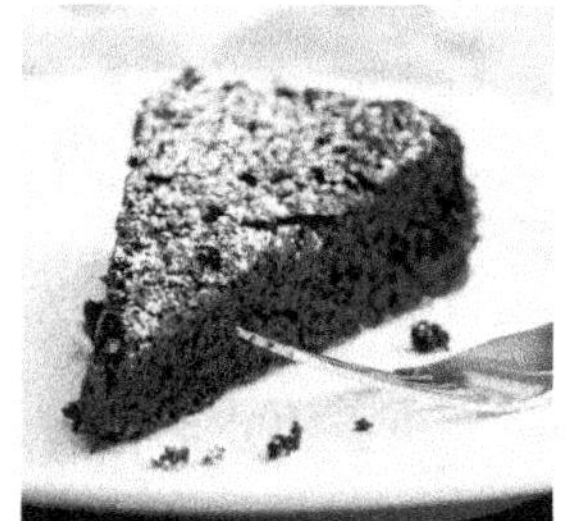

This easy-to-make chocolate cake is dark, moist, rich—and only dirties one bowl! Not quite as easy as boxed cake mixes, but those often contain trans fats. Our simple "from scratch" recipe gives you a home-baked cake with healthful canola oil and whole-wheat flour.

Ingredients 12 servings

¾ cup plus 2 tablespoons whole-wheat pastry flour, (see Ingredient Note)

½ cup granulated sugar

⅔ cup Unsweetened cocoa powder

1 teaspoon baking powder

1 teaspoon baking soda

¼ teaspoon salt

½ cup nonfat buttermilk,

½ cup packed light brown sugar

1 large egg, lightly beaten

2 tablespoons canola oil

1 teaspoon vanilla extract

½ cup hot strong black coffee

Confectioners' sugar, for dusting

Preparation

Active

25 m

Ready In

1 h 5 min

Preheat oven to 350°F. Coat a 9-inch round cake pan with cooking spray. Line the pan with a circle of wax paper.

Whisk flour, granulated sugar, cocoa, baking powder, baking soda and salt in a large bowl. Add buttermilk, brown sugar, egg, oil and vanilla. Beat with an electric mixer on medium speed for 2 minutes. Add hot coffee and beat to blend. (The batter will be quite thin.) Pour the batter into the prepared pan.

Bake the cake until a skewer inserted in the center comes out clean, 30 to 35 minutes. Cool in the pan on a wire rack for 10 minutes; remove from the pan, peel off the wax paper and let cool completely. Dust the top with confectioners' sugar before slicing.

Ingredient Note: Whole-wheat pastry flour, lower in protein than regular whole-wheat flour, has less gluten-forming potential, making it a better choice for tender baked goods. You can find it in the natural-foods section of large supermarkets and natural-foods stores. Store in the freezer.

Tip: No buttermilk? You can use buttermilk powder prepared according to package directions. Or make "sour milk": mix 1 tablespoon lemon juice or vinegar to 1 cup milk.

Nutrition information

Per serving: 139 calories; 3 g fat(0 g sat); 2 g fiber; 27 g carbohydrates; 2 g protein; 3 mcg folate; 16 mg cholesterol; 19 g sugars; 18 g added sugars; 22 IU vitamin A; 0 mg vitamin C; 38 mg calcium; 1 mg iron; 212 mg sodium; 63 mg potassium

Apricot-Walnut Cereal Bars

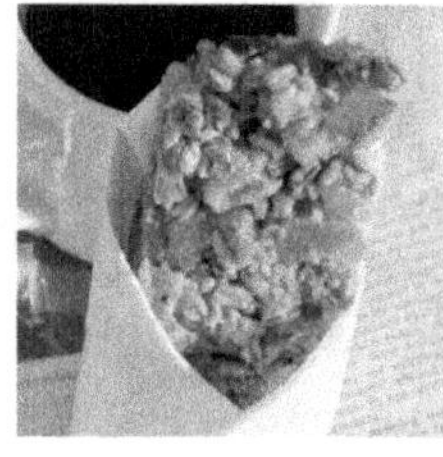

Crisp and chewy, this bar is a good-for-you alternative to store-bought cereal bars. The secret ingredient, silken tofu, will give your day a protein-packed start. The recipe also works with other fruit-and-nut combinations.

Ingredients 16 servings

3 cups old-fashioned rolled oats

½ cup chopped walnuts, (about 2 ounces)

3 cups unsweetened puffed-grain cereal, such as Kashi

2 cups chopped dried apricots

¼ cup all-purpose flour

½ teaspoon salt

12 ounces silken tofu, drained (about 1? cups)

1 large egg

½ cup canola oil

1 cup honey

1 tablespoon vanilla extract

2 tablespoons freshly grated lemon zest

Preparation

Active

30 m

Ready In

2 h

Preheat oven to 350°F. Coat a large (15¼-by-10¼-inch) jellyroll-style pan with cooking spray.

Spread oats and walnuts on a baking sheet with sides. Bake until fragrant and light golden, 8 to 10 minutes. Transfer to a large bowl and add puffed cereal, dried apricots, flour and salt; stir to combine.

Meanwhile, puree tofu, egg, oil, honey, vanilla and lemon zest in a food processor or blender until smooth, scraping down the sides as needed. Make a well in the center of the oat mixture; fold in the tofu mixture until combined. Spread evenly in the prepared pan.

Bake until firm in the center and golden brown, 35 to 40 minutes. Let cool completely in the pan on a wire rack before cutting into bars with a sharp knife.

Make Ahead Tip: Individually wrap in plastic and keep at room temperature for up to 5 days or freeze for up to 1 month. Thaw at room temperature or remove plastic, wrap in a paper towel and defrost according to your microwave's directions.

Easy cleanup: Dessert pans can be a headache to clean. Skip the soaking and scrubbing by lining your pan with parchment paper before you bake.

Nutrition information

Serving size: 1 bar

Per serving: 286 calories; 11 g fat(1 g sat); 4 g fiber; 44 g carbohydrates; 5 g protein; 11 mcg folate; 12 mg cholesterol; 25 g sugars; 208 IU vitamin A; 1 mg vitamin C; 31 mg calcium; 2 mg iron; 98 mg sodium; 289 mg potassium

Ginger Crinkle Cookies

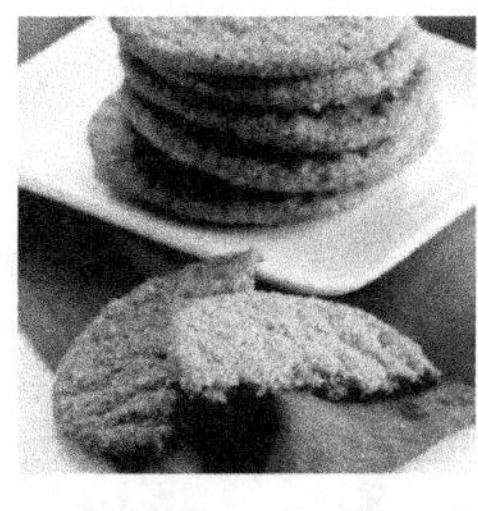

Cynthia Farr-Weinfeld, a hypnotherapist and writer, started improving the nutritional profile of a friend's mother's ginger cookie recipe by substituting whole-wheat pastry flour for all-purpose flour and canola oil for shortening. "Experiment with these cookies," she advises, "as they taste great either slightly underdone or crispy." She calls them "the q uickest cookies you'll ever bake."

Ingredients 1 serving

⅔ cup canola oil

1½ cups turbinado sugar, divided (see Tip)

1 large egg

4 tablespoons molasses

2 cups sifted whole-wheat pastry flour

2 teaspoons baking soda

1¼ teaspoons ground cinnamon

1¼ teaspoons ground ginger

¼ teaspoon sea salt

Preparation

Active

10 m

Ready In

1 h

Preheat oven to 350°F.

Mix oil and 1 cup sugar in a large bowl until combined. Beat in egg until combined. Stir in molasses until evenly incorporated. Sift flour, baking soda, cinnamon, ginger and salt over the wet ingredients and stir until just combined.

Put the remaining ½ cup sugar in a small bowl. Roll the dough into 1-inch balls and roll each ball in the sugar before placing 2 inches apart on an ungreased baking sheet. Do not flatten.

Bake the cookies until set, but still soft when gently touched, 10 to 12 minutes. Transfer to a wire rack to cool.

Make Ahead Tip: Store in an airtight container at room temperature for up to 5 days.

Tip: Turbinado sugar is steam-cleaned raw cane sugar. It's coarse-grained and light brown in color, with a slight molasses flavor. The coarse texture adds great crunch when used in baking. Find it in the natural-foods section of large supermarkets or at natural-foods stores.

Storage smarts: To extend the life of your baked goods, store them in an airtight container in a single layer or between layers of parchment paper to prevent sticking.

Nutrition information

Per serving: 103 calories; 5 g fat(0 g sat); 1 g fiber; 15 g carbohydrates; 1 g protein; 1 mcg folate; 5 mg cholesterol; 10 g sugars; 9 g added sugars;

8 IU vitamin A; 0 mg vitamin C; 7 mg calcium; 0 mg iron; 93 mg sodium; 38 mg potassium

Boot Tracks

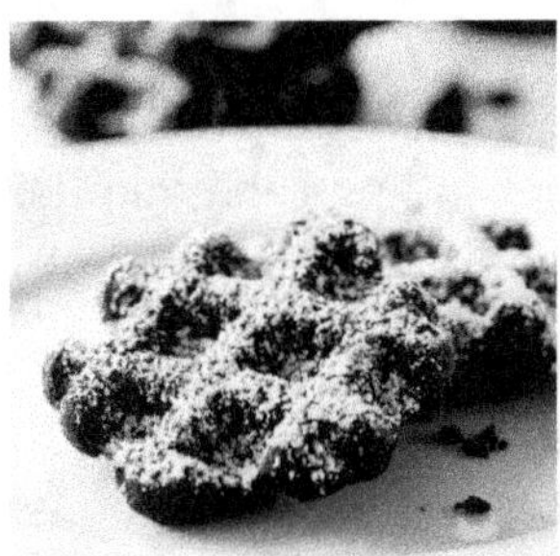

Patti Anderson, a professional q uilter, had never entered a cooking contest before she took our challenge. This q uick, no-fuss, chewy chocolate cookie is made on your waffle iron. No need to haul out the big mixer, you can mix the batter with a small hand mixer or even by hand. Kids love these!

Ingredients 1 serving

½ cup salted butter

⅔ cup granulated sugar

2 large eggs

1 teaspoon vanilla extract

1 cup whole-wheat pastry flour

6 tablespoons cocoa powder

2 tablespoons canola oil

½ teaspoon espresso powder, (optional)

Confectioners' sugar, for dusting

Preparation

Active

30 min

Ready In

30 min

Preheat a nonstick (not Belgian) waffle iron.

Cream butter and sugar in a medium bowl. Beat in eggs and vanilla. Add flour, cocoa powder, oil and espresso powder (if using). Beat until thoroughly combined.

Drop the batter by rounded teaspoonfuls about 1 inch apart onto the preheated ungreased waffle iron. (To avoid burnt fingers, use two spoons, one to scoop and one to scrape dough onto the waffle iron.) Close and cook until the cookies are puffed and cooked through, 1 to 1½ minutes. Waffle irons vary, so watch closely and don't let the cookies get too dark. Transfer to a wire rack to cool until just warm. Dust the cookies with confectioners' sugar while still slightly warm (see Variations).

Variations: Instead of confectioners' sugar, drizzle cooled cookies with melted bittersweet and/or white chocolate. Or make a peppermint drizzle: Mix 1 cup confectioners' sugar, 4 teaspoons water and ¼ teaspoon peppermint extract; add natural green food coloring, if desired.

Make Ahead Tip: Store in an airtight container for up to 1 day. Dust with additional confectioners' sugar just before serving.

Decorate on parchment: When adding finishing touches to your cookies or cakes, place them on a large sheet of parchment paper before you decorate. The paper catches the excess, making cleanup a breeze.

Nutrition information

Serving size: 1 cookie

Per serving: 63 calories; 4 g fat(2 g sat); 1 g fiber; 7 g carbohydrates; 1 g protein; 2 mcg folate; 17 mg cholesterol; 4 g sugars; 4 g added sugars; 94 IU vitamin A; 0 mg vitamin C; 4 mg calcium; 0 mg iron; 24 mg sodium; 18 mg potassium

Warm Chocolate Pudding

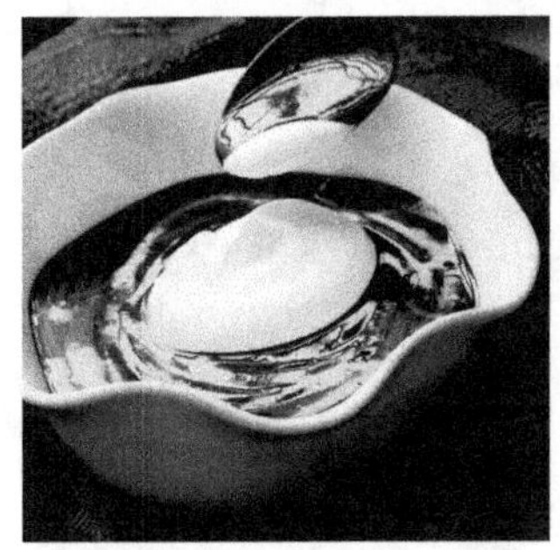

This warm pudding has a marvelous deep chocolaty flavor, but it's low in fat and super-quick to make. Don't skimp on the quality of cocoa with this one—treat yourself to the good stuff.

Ingredients 6 servings

1 large egg

2¼ cups nonfat or low-fat milk, divided

⅔ cup sugar, divided

⅔ teaspoon salt

⅔ cup unsweetened cocoa powder

2 tablespoons cornstarch

1 teaspoon vanilla extract

Preparation

Active

20 min

Ready In

20 min

Lightly beat egg with a fork in a medium bowl.

Combine 1½ cups milk, ? cup sugar and salt in a medium saucepan; bring to a simmer over medium heat, stirring occasionally.

Meanwhile, whisk the remaining ? cup sugar, cocoa and cornstarch in a medium bowl. Whisk in the remaining ¾ cup milk until blended. Whisk the simmering milk mixture into the cocoa mixture. Pour the mixture back into the pan and bring to a simmer over medium heat, whisking constantly, until thickened and glossy, about 3 minutes. Remove from heat.

Whisk about 1 cup of the hot cocoa mixture into the beaten egg. Return the egg mixture to the pan and cook over medium-low heat, whisking constantly, until steaming and thickened, about 2 minutes. (Do not boil.) Whisk in vanilla. Serve warm.

Make Ahead Tip: Pour the pudding into a bowl and place a piece of plastic wrap directly on the surface. Refrigerate for up to 3 days; serve cold.

Nutrition information

Per serving: 164 calories; 2 g fat(1 g sat); 4 g fiber; 35 g carbohydrates; 6 g protein; 12 mcg folate; 33 mg cholesterol; 27 g sugars; 22 g added sugars; 59 IU vitamin A; 0 mg vitamin C; 129 mg calcium; 2 mg iron; 101 mg sodium; 302 mg potassium

Mediterranean Dinner

Skillet Gnocchi with Chard & White Beans

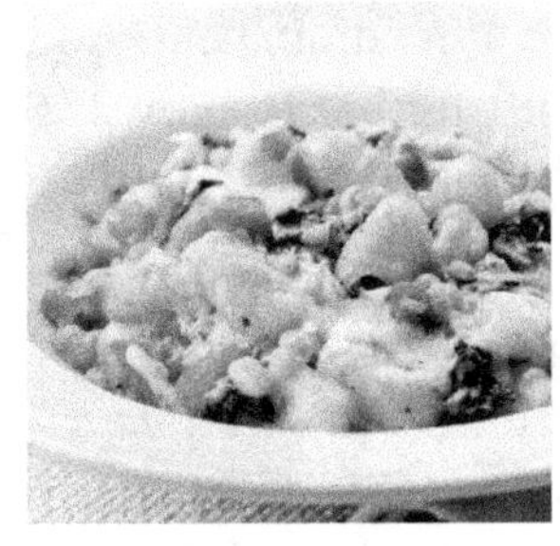

In this one-skillet supper, we toss dark leafy greens, diced tomatoes and white beans with gnocchi and top it all with gooey mozzarella. Serve with a mixed green salad with vinaigrette.

Ingredients 6 servings

1 tablespoon plus 1 teaspoon extra-virgin olive oil, divided

1 16-ounce package shelf-stable gnocchi, (see Tip)

1 medium yellow onion, thinly sliced

4 cloves garlic, minced

½ cup water

6 cups chopped chard leaves, (about 1 small bunch) or spinach

1 15-ounce can diced tomatoes with Italian seasonings

1 15-ounce can white beans, rinsed

¼ teaspoon freshly ground pepper

½ cup shredded part-skim mozzarella cheese

¼ cup finely shredded Parmesan cheese

Preparation

Active

30 min

Ready In

30 min

Heat 1 tablespoon oil in a large nonstick skillet over medium heat. Add gnocchi and cook, stirring often, until plumped and starting to brown, 5 to 7 minutes. Transfer to a bowl.

Add the remaining 1 teaspoon oil and onion to the pan and cook, stirring, over medium heat, for 2 minutes. Stir in garlic and water. Cover and cook until the onion is soft, 4 to 6 minutes. Add chard (or spinach) and cook, stirring, until starting to wilt, 1 to 2 minutes. Stir in tomatoes, beans and pepper and bring to a simmer. Stir in the gnocchi and sprinkle with mozzarella and Parmesan. Cover and cook until the cheese is melted and the sauce is bubbling, about 3 minutes.

Tip: Look for shelf-stable gnocchi near other pasta in the Italian section of most supermarkets.

Nutrition information

Serving size: 1 cup

Per serving: 326 calories; 7 g fat(2 g sat); 6 g fiber; 56 g carbohydrates; 14 g protein; 60 mcg folate; 9 mg cholesterol; 5 g sugars; 0 g added sugars; 2,724 IU vitamin A; 28 mg vitamin C; 191 mg calcium; 4 mg iron; 610 mg sodium; 366 mg potassium

Easy Salmon Cakes

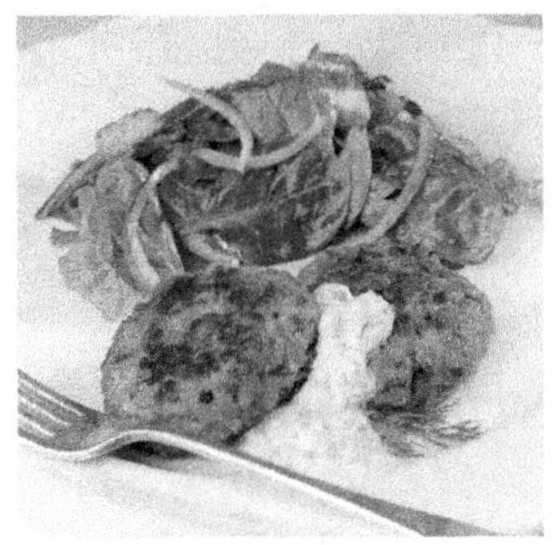

If you are trying to boost your intake of omega-3s, try this simple favorite. It is a great way to use convenient canned (or leftover) salmon. The tangy dill sauce provides a tart balance.

Ingredients 4 servings

3 teaspoons extra-virgin olive oil, divided

1 small onion, finely chopped

Onions Red

1 stalk celery, finely diced

2 tablespoons chopped fresh parsley

15 ounces canned salmon, drained, or 1½ cups cooked salmon

1 large egg, lightly beaten

1½ teaspoons Dijon mustard

1¾ cups fresh whole-wheat breadcrumbs, (see Tip)

½ teaspoon freshly ground pepper

Creamy Dill Sauce, (recipe follows)

1 lemon, cut into wedges

Preparation

Active

30 min

Ready In

45 min

Preheat oven to 450°F. Coat a baking sheet with cooking spray.

Heat 1½ teaspoons oil in a large nonstick skillet over medium-high heat. Add onion and celery; cook, stirring, until softened, about 3 minutes. Stir in parsley; remove from the heat.

Place salmon in a medium bowl. Flake apart with a fork; remove any bones and skin. Add egg and mustard; mix well. Add the onion mixture, breadcrumbs and pepper; mix well. Shape the mixture into 8 patties, about 2½ inches wide.

Heat remaining 1½ teaspoons oil in the pan over medium heat. Add 4 patties and cook until the undersides are golden, 2 to 3 minutes. Using a wide spatula, turn them over onto the prepared baking sheet. Repeat with the remaining patties.

Bake the salmon cakes until golden on top and heated through, 15 to 20 minutes. Meanwhile, prepare Creamy Dill Sauce. Serve salmon cakes with sauce and lemon wedges.

Make Ahead Tip: Prepare through step 3. Cover and refrigerate for up to 8 hours.

To make fresh breadcrumbs: Trim crusts from firm sandwich bread. Tear the bread into pieces and process in a food processor until coarse crumbs form. One slice makes about ? cup.

Easy cleanup: Recipes that req uire cooking spray can leave behind a sticky residue that can be hard to clean. To save time and keep your baking sheet looking fresh, line it with a layer of foil before you apply the cooking spray.

Nutrition information

Per serving: 350 calories; 14 g fat(1 g sat); 6 g fiber; 26 g carbohydrates; 34 g protein; 26 mcg folate; 126 mg cholesterol; 5 g sugars; 419 IU vitamin A; 7 mg vitamin C; 60 mg calcium; 2 mg iron; 761 mg sodium; 169 mg potassium

Chicken Breasts with Mushroom Cream Sauce

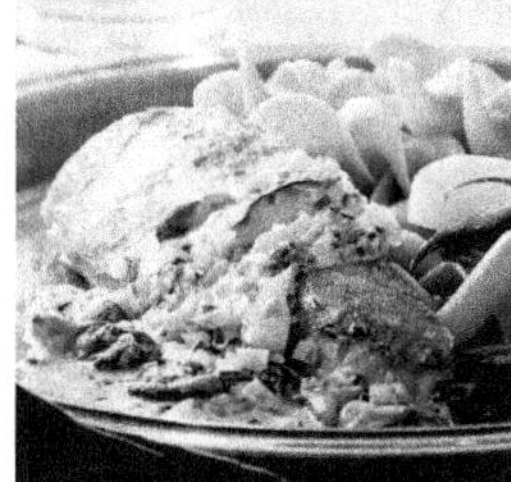 The secret to a good cream sauce is always the same: not too much cream or it can be overpowering, masking the more delicate flavors. Here it contains a bountiful amount of mushrooms and is served over chicken breasts.

Ingredients 2 servings

2 5-ounce boneless, skinless chicken breasts, trimmed and tenders removed (see Tip)

½ teaspoon freshly ground pepper

¼ teaspoon salt

1 tablespoon canola oil

1 medium shallot, minced

1 cup thinly sliced shiitake mushroom caps

2 tablespoons dry vermouth, or dry white wine

¼ cup reduced-sodium chicken broth

2 tablespoons heavy cream

2 tablespoons minced fresh chives, or scallion greens

Preparation

Active

30 min

Ready In

30 min

Season chicken with pepper and salt on both sides.

Heat oil in a medium skillet over medium heat. Add the chicken and cook, turning once or twice and adjusting the heat to prevent burning, until brown and an instant-read thermometer inserted into the thickest part registers 165°F, 12 to 16 minutes. Transfer to a plate and tent with foil to keep warm.

Add shallot to the pan and cook, stirring, until fragrant, about 30 seconds. Add mushrooms; cook, stirring occasionally, until tender, about 2 minutes. Pour in vermouth (or wine); simmer until almost evaporated, scraping up any browned bits, about 1 minute. Pour in broth and cook until reduced by half, 1 to 2 minutes. Stir in cream and chives (or scallions); return to a simmer. Return the chicken to the pan, turn to coat with sauce and cook until heated through, about 1 minute.

It's difficult to find an individual chicken breast small enough for one portion. Removing the thin strip of meat from the underside of a 5-ounce breast—the "tender"—removes about 1 ounce of meat and yields a perfect 4-ounce portion. Wrap and freeze the tenders and when you have gathered enough, use them in a stir-fry or for oven-baked chicken fingers.

Nutrition information

Serving size: 3 oz. chicken & ¼ cup sauce

Per serving: 274 calories; 15 g fat(5 g sat); 1 g fiber; 5 g carbohydrates; 25 g protein; 19 mcg folate; 83 mg cholesterol; 2 g sugars; 0 g added sugars; 548 IU vitamin A; 4 mg vitamin C; 33 mg calcium; 1 mg iron; 425 mg sodium; 403 mg potassium

Broccoli-Cheese Chowder

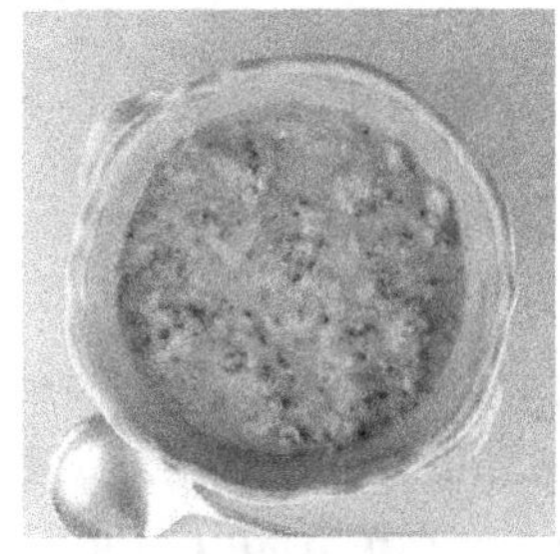 This satisfying remake of broccoli chowder benefits from the creamy texture of cooked potatoes and smooth, tangy reduced-fat sour cream instead of getting its richness from as much as a cup each of cream and cheese. Not only is the flavor vibrant, but a single serving gives you over half of the daily recommendation for vitamin C.

Ingredients 6 servings

1 tablespoon extra-virgin olive oil

1 large onion, chopped

1 large carrot, diced

2 stalks celery, diced

1 large potato, peeled and diced

2 cloves garlic, minced

1 tablespoon all-purpose flour

½ teaspoon dry mustard

¾ cayenne pepper

2 14-ounce cans vegetable broth, or reduced-sodium chicken broth

8 ounces broccoli crowns, (see Ingredient Note), cut into 1-inch pieces, stems and florets separated

1 cup shredded reduced-fat Cheddar cheese

½ cup reduced-fat sour cream

¾ teaspoon salt

Preparation

Active

45 min

Ready In

1 h 5 min

Heat oil in a Dutch oven or large saucepan over medium-high heat. Add onion, carrot and celery; cook, stirring often, until the onion and celery soften, 5 to 6 minutes. Add potato and garlic; cook, stirring, for 2 minutes. Stir in flour, dry mustard and cayenne; cook, stirring often, for 2 minutes.

Add broth and broccoli stems; bring to a boil. Cover and reduce heat to medium. Simmer, stirring occasionally, for 10 minutes. Stir in florets; simmer, covered, until the broccoli is tender, about 10 minutes more. Transfer 2 cups of the chowder to a bowl and mash; return to the pan.

Stir in Cheddar and sour cream; cook over medium heat, stirring, until the cheese is melted and the chowder is heated through, about 2 minutes. Season with salt.

Make Ahead Tip: Prepare through Step 2. Cover and refrigerate for up to 2 days or freeze for up to 2 months.

Ingredient note: Most supermarkets sell broccoli crowns, which are the tops of the bunches, with the stalks cut off. Although crowns are more expensive than entire bunches, they are convenient and there is considerably less waste.

Nutrition information

Serving size: 1 cup

Per serving: 199 calories; 9 g fat(4 g sat); 4 g fiber; 23 g carbohydrates; 9 g protein; 41 mcg folate; 21 mg cholesterol; 5 g sugars; 2,634 IU vitamin

A; 36 mg vitamin C; 331 mg calcium; 1 mg iron; 623 mg sodium; 436 mg potassium

Chilaq uiles Casserole

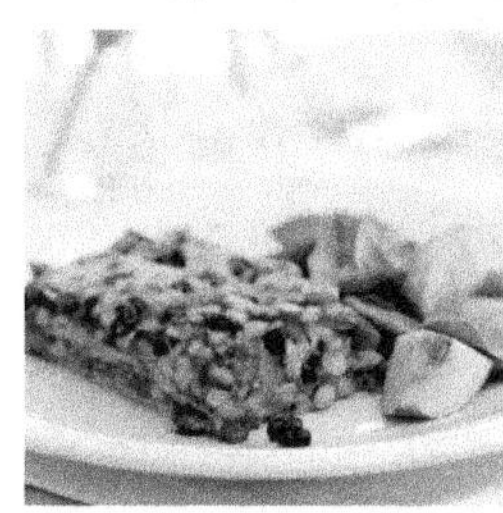

Ingredients 1 serving

1 tablespoon canola oil

1 medium onion, diced

1 medium zucchini, grated

1 19-ounce can black beans, rinsed

1 14-ounce can diced tomatoes, drained

1½ cups corn, frozen (thawed) or fresh

1 teaspoon ground cumin

½ teaspoon salt

12 corn tortillas, q uartered

1 19-ounce can mild red or green enchilada sauce

1¼ cups shredded reduced-fat Cheddar cheese

Preparation

Active

20 min

Ready In

45 min

Preheat oven to 400°F. Lightly coat a 9-by-13-inch baking pan with cooking spray.

Heat oil in a large nonstick skillet over medium-high heat. Add onion and cook, stirring often, until starting to brown, about 5 minutes. Stir in zucchini, beans, tomatoes, corn, cumin and salt and cook, stirring occasionally, until the vegetables are heated through, about 3 minutes.

Scatter half the tortilla pieces in the pan. Top with half the vegetable mixture, half the enchilada sauce and half the cheese. Repeat with one more layer of tortillas, vegetables, sauce and cheese. Cover with foil.

Bake the casserole for 15 minutes. Remove the foil and continue baking until the casserole is bubbling around the edges and the cheese is melted, about 10 minutes more.

Make Ahead Tip: Prepare through Step 3 and refrigerate for up to 1 day.

Nutrition information

Serving size: 1 piece

Per serving: 238 calories; 10 g fat(5 g sat); 6 g fiber; 30 g carbohydrates; 9 g protein; 39 mcg folate; 23 mg cholesterol; 4 g sugars; 0 g added sugars; 690 IU vitamin A; 16 mg vitamin C; 120 mg calcium; 2 mg iron; 369 mg sodium; 362 mg potassium

CONCLUSION

Cooking is great fun for many people. It can foster relationships and

improve family bonding. In order cook great dishes, you must make sure

that you have followed the cooking recipe closely.